S.M.I.L.Y.
Sensory Motor Integration & Learning with Yoga

April Merrilee

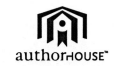

1663 LIBERTY DRIVE, SUITE 200
BLOOMINGTON, INDIANA 47403
(800) 839-8640
www.AuthorHouse.com

© 2006 April Merrilee. All rights reserved.

No part of this book may be reproduced, stored in a retrieval system, or transmitted by any means without the written permission of the author.

First published by AuthorHouse 2/16/2006

ISBN: 1-4208-7422-5

Library of Congress Control Number: 2005907795

Printed in the United States of America
Bloomington, Indiana

This book is printed on acid-free paper.

1) The S.M.I.L.Y. program is a facet of the company known as Stream of Life Therapeutics LLC, which is owned and operated solely by April Merrilee. All transactions and events related to the S.M.I.L.Y. program therefore operate under the auspices of this limited liability company.

2) The S.M.I.L.Y. program is based on the use of yoga postures that are basic and safe to perform without any previous yoga experience. The practice of yoga, like any physical exercise program, contains inherent risks and could result in injury if not performed carefully by each individual. Children should be instructed and supervised for safety. The author of this book hereby releases any responsibility or liability for any injuries incurred from the practice of the S.M.I.L.Y. program. Please consult your health care provider regarding any safety or health concerns.

3) The S.M.I.L.Y. lesson materials (drawings and worksheets) provided in Section 8 are reproducible for use with children only. No part of this book may be used for the purpose of presentations, workshops or resale of any kind.

ACKNOWLEDGEMENTS

I am so grateful for the support and generosity of so many wonderful friends and acquaintances (many of whom became friends during this process)! I extend the deepest thanks to DeAnna and Joe Hoyle who opened their work space and their hearts to me without limitation so that I could learn how to draw stick figures using the Corel Draw program on their computer. Whew! I also want to express my gratitude toward Brad and Felicia Meyer for loaning me their wonderful camera and use of their software for processing the digital photographs in this text. Of equal importance are the families and children who allowed me to take their photographs - you are all such beautiful stars! Thanks to the various teachers and therapists who have assisted in the development of the SMILY program in so many ways: Marjorie, Tammy, Amilia and most especially Diann. You are well remembered. I am also greatly appreciative of the editorial services so freely given by Sue, Sharon, Kathy and Sky. Thanks to my loving parents, Maxine and Sandy Sanderson, for helping me believe I really could do this my way! And, as ever, I am thankful for the never ending support of my love, L.D. (Is it 3:00?)

The most excellent yoga models in these photographs are:

Ella Blechman	25 months	Sierra Karas	5 years
Alexandria Karas	30 months	Averie Lynch	6 years
Dylan Manzanares	33 months	Gavin Ross	7 years
Sarah Ross	4 years	Marley Gabel	7 years
Bea Polczynski	4 years	Carter Walsh	10 years
William Meyer	5 years		

Table of Contents

SECTION ONE: What is S.M.I.L.Y.? — 1

SECTION TWO: Yoga as Sensory Motor Integration — 6
Definition and Benefits of SI
Guiding Principles and Adaptive Responses

SECTION THREE: Research and Literature Review — 16
Yoga for Children
Movement, Brain Development and Learning
Music and Childhood Development
Supporting Literacy Skills

SECTION FOUR: Components of Learning and the SMILY Approach — 31
Sensory – Motor Components
Handwriting and Literacy Skills
Multiple Intelligences

SECTION FIVE: In the School Setting — 42
Multi-disciplinary Approach
Least Restrictive Environment (LRE)
General Education Benchmarks

SECTION SIX Special Education: Therapists & Teachers — 51
Individualized Education Plans (IEP's)
Therapy Goals: OT, PT, SLP

SECTION SEVEN: How to Teach Children Breathing, Relaxation & Postures — 58
Breathing, Relaxation and Poses

SECTION EIGHT: S.M.I.L.Y. Routines & Materials — 67
Directions for SMILY Functional Activities
Lesson Materials – Reproducible for use with children (only!)

SECTION NINE: Additional Information — 279
About the Author
SMILY Workshops and CD Soundtrack

LIST OF TABLES

Table 1:	Shared Benefits of Yoga and SI treatment	9
Table 2:	Multiple Sensory Channels	11
Table 3:	Principles of Sensory Integrative Treatment	12
Table 4:	Adaptive responses facilitated by SMILY	13
Table 5:	Research on Yoga for Children	18
Table 6:	Learning in the Brain	23
Table 7:	Theories of Brain Development	25
Table 8:	Music and Childhood Development	28
Table 9:	Literacy Skill Building	29
Table 10:	Sensory and Motor Components of Learning	33
Table 11:	Motor Components of Handwriting	36
Table 12:	Handwriting Models of Intervention	37
Table 13:	Encouraging Literacy	38
Table 14:	Components of Literacy Skills	39
Table 15:	Multiple Intelligences	41
Table 16:	Least Restrictive Environment	45
Table 17:	Language Arts Benchmarks	47
Table 18:	Mathematics Benchmarks	48
Table 19:	Physical Education Benchmarks	49
Table 20:	Arts Performance Benchmarks	50
Table 21:	Sample Therapy Goals for OT, PT & SLP	54
Table 22:	Therapy Log Table	57
Table 23:	Benefits of Breathing	59
Table 24:	Benefits of Relaxation	60

SECTION ONE: What is S.M.I.L.Y.?

Sensory Motor Integration & Learning with Yoga

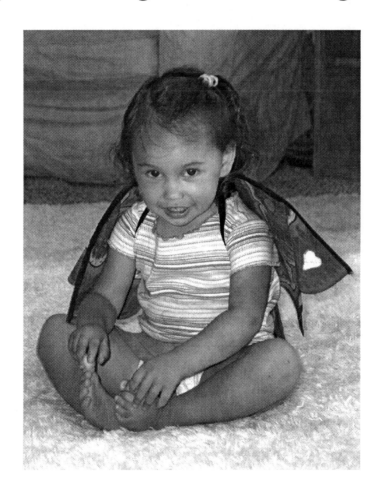

SMILY arose out of my desire to share the benefits of yoga with children in my role as a pediatric Occupational Therapist working in a school setting. I wanted to provide children, therapists and teachers with a **fun and unique** way of enhancing the development of skills needed for success at school. I also knew that the use of yoga could be justified as an effective method to stimulate learning while supporting basic educational requirements. My hope is that you find this book very user-friendly. I have tried my best to include everything you need to incorporate the SMILY program into your weekly lessons and/or treatment planning. Hopefully this book will serve as a clear guide for introducing music and movement, in the form of yoga, to the children in your life.

SMILY is most appropriate for children ages 3 - 9 in the pre-school and elementary school settings. It can be taught by Occupational, Speech and Physical Therapists. SMILY can also be offered by P.E. teachers, Regular Ed teachers and Resource teachers working in Special Education. Parents, clinicians and caregivers can also successfully use the SMILY program in their settings. SMILY is both fun and flexible; it can be easily modified to meet the needs of children with varying abilities and across multiple placements. Within its flexibility, SMILY offers a very structured format, making it an easy method of service delivery for therapists and teachers. It provides a consistent, detailed structure for treatment/lesson planning. Teachers can observe the educational benchmarks being met in the process, and children are able to see and enjoy their own progress as they advance through the music and movement routines.

The SMILY program consists of eight distinct yoga routines paired with music in the form of children's songs. The characters in the songs are the names of the yoga poses. There are 8 poses in each routine, always presented in the same order to go along with the song lyrics. These poses are taught through the use of stick figure drawings, demonstration and hands-on assistance as needed. The use of stick figure drawings is a central component of the SMILY approach. For each session, the sequence of 8 postures is hung along the wall in order from left to right at eye level for the children. All the drawings and materials needed for the entire SMILY program are included in this book, and reproducible for use with children.

Imitation of posture from the stick figures is a powerful method for learning important concepts of body image, body scheme, motor planning, spatial relations and sequencing skills. Modeling of the postures by adults further supports the development of complex sensory-motor integrative skills. For children who have greater difficulty with motor planning or balance, a touch here or there can be a very helpful way to help them orient their bodies in space. Please see the section entitled, "How to Teach Children" for details on guiding students through the SMILY routines.

Vocabulary and reading skills are strengthened in many ways, most especially through the integration of auditory and visual input. The name of each posture is printed above all the stick figure drawings, embedded in the lyrics of each song, and built into fine motor and visual perceptual activities that follow each routine. The songs are first presented in a story format, helping the children initially to learn the words and later to repeat the story back to us independently. Singing helps promote components of literacy skills such as sequencing, rhythm, repetition and memorization. These skills are also enhanced through the educationally relevant activities or "lessons" that are included in every session. The SMILY program is designed to enhance the components involved in developing the basic literacy skills of reading and writing! Look to the section entitled, "Components of Learning & the SMILY Approach" for specific details.

Deep breathing or belly breathing is an essential part of the program, taught as a learned skill and woven into the practice. I emphasize the importance of starting each session with belly breathing in a back lying position to help the children focus their attention. Each session also includes the very important aspect of trained relaxation practice following the yoga poses. Suggestions for teaching breathing and relaxation to children, and the benefits, are included later in this book, in the "How to Teach Children" section.

Following relaxation, the children move on to a series of structured, functional tasks that focus on the development of visual motor, visual perceptual, fine motor and language skills. The movement and music serve as sensory motor stimulation, in preparation for the "adaptive response" of these higher level functional activities at the end of each session. These structured activities comprise the "SMILY Lessons" that are outlined in more detail later. These lessons were designed to support curriculum based benchmarks. A review of your state educational standards will show how SMILY can be used to reinforce specific academic areas. For a general idea of how the SMILY program supports educational benchmarks, please refer to the section, "In the School Setting". This section also includes sample Occupational, Physical and Speech Therapy goals for IEP's.

The SMILY Lessons generated by each routine can be introduced gradually as the children learn the movements and language associated with the yoga poses. Each routine is linked to a structured series of 10 specific activities or lesson. Therefore, each routine can be practiced for a number of weeks as the group progresses through the lessons. As such, the entire SMILY program of nine routines provides enough educationally relevant lessons to fill an entire academic year!

Depending upon frequency of sessions, you may focus on one routine per month or stretch a single routine out for six or even eight weeks. This also depends upon the functional levels of the students in your groups. Some children will move more rapidly through the music, movement, and activities than others. The program leaves room for flexibility with regard to scheduling and progressing through each routine. A full SMILY session can take place in as little as 30 minutes, once per week. Just this amount of time will provide some wonderful benefits. A longer session of 45 minutes is even better, and two sessions per week is ideal! Take what is best for your students and give them the components that they really need the most. Feel free to make the SMILY program your own – individualize it as needed to fit the requirements of your children and your schedule!

Yoga for children is quite different than yoga for adults. With children we are not trying to perform all the postures perfectly or to achieve "polished" looking poses. Yes, we want them to practice the postures safely. And yes, we want them to practice with enough accuracy to promote strength, flexibility, balance and coordination. (See "How to Teach Children".) Aside from these considerations, we mostly want them to enjoy the experience of learning yoga: the breathing, the poses, and the relaxation. We make it fun by pairing the movement with music. And we make it educational by including activities for language development, handwriting and literacy skills.

Perhaps most importantly, by introducing the basic concepts of yoga at an early age, we are planting the seed for practicing later in life. I hope that through this introduction to yoga, the children I work with will be more interested in a healthy lifestyle approach as adults. They will already know what yoga is and how it helps them. I like to think that years from now, one of my students will feel comfortable joining an adult yoga class because he will remember doing it with us in school as a child. He'll say, "I know how to do yoga - we used to do it with Miss April!".

SECTION TWO:
Yoga as Sensory Motor Integration

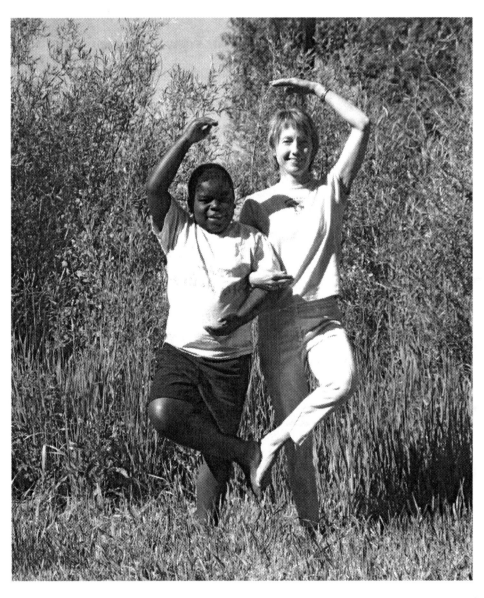

Definition of S.I.

The ever growing field of Sensory Integration exists as both a theory of neurological functions (as they relate to behavior) as well as an on-going process of the human body and mind interacting with the environment. Traditionally, three types of sensory input comprise the cornerstone of the SI approach. These are: tactile, proprioception and vestibular stimulation.

Tactile is our sense of touch, and is especially regulated through sensitive areas such as the hand, feet and head. Proprioception is an umbrella term for the sense of body position and is involved in body awareness in space, planning and coordinating movements, and emotional security and confidence. Proprioceptive input is sent to the brain through receptors in the muscles, joints, tendons and ligaments. The vestibular system is comprised of sense receptors in the inner ear as well as the fibers of Cranial Nerve VIII (Vestibulocochlear) connected to those structures.

Sensory Integration theory teaches us that the vestibular system can have the greatest impact on both the modulation of sensory input as well as the development of all types of skills. The vestibular system is related to the regulation of muscle tone, balance, motor control, postural control, visual space perception, visual-motor control, auditory language skills and attention.

As such, Sensory Integration involves an interpretation of sensory-motor integration within the global context of being human: of receiving and processing sensory input and producing desired "out-come" behavior or result. In this big picture view, sensory-motor integration is a continuous, fundamental constant of living and being for humans of all ages. Seeing the children we work with as whole and complete beings is a central aspect of the SMILY approach. Providing them with purposeful, multi-sensory based activities has been the objective of therapists for years. In this regard, SMILY is indeed a process of sensory-motor integration.

This book will not cover more precise neurological elements or the efficacy of Sensory Integration theory and treatment. These points are well documented and a vast array of literature is available to readers wishing to deepen their knowledge. My intention is to show how the SMILY program, as a blend of music and movement, supports the principles, components and functions of a sensory-motor approach to therapy. It is, however, necessary to review some basics in the field of Sensory Integration in order to highlight the SMILY approach. I have simplified much of this information into the form of tables and lists so that this book is "user-friendly."

So how can we view the SMILY program as a process of sensory-motor integration? First, we must have some idea of what Sensory Integration is and why it is important to provide sensory-motor experiences to children as they develop. For this we turn to the seminal work of Dr. A. Jean Ayres, the Occupational Therapist who first discovered and developed the theory and treatment techniques known as Sensory Integration. In her book, <u>Sensory Integration and the Child</u> (1979), she writes:

> Sensory integration is the organization of sensation for use. Our senses give us information about the physical conditions of our body and the environment around us...Countless bits of sensory information enter our brain at every moment, not only from our eyes and ears, but also from every place in our bodies...You can think of sensations as "food for the brain"; they provide the energy and knowledge needed to direct the body and mind. But without well organized sensory processes, sensations cannot be digested and nourish the brain.

Sensory integration involves the brain's ability to organize sensation from the body and from the environment in order to use the body (and mind) effectively. Constant communication between the brain, the environment and the body involves all parts of the nervous system: cortex and sub-cortical brain/ brainstem; spinal cord; autonomic nervous system for regulating bodily functions and the peripheral nervous system for processing sensory input and motor output.

All this information comes into the brain, is perceived and processed, and then we are able to produce a motor or behavioral outcome. This is sometimes referred to as a feedback loop that produces an "adaptive response" which is a functional behavior. The highest functional outcomes (adaptive responses) are evident when the sensory-motor system is organized and working optimally. We will take a much closer look at the role of adaptive responses later in this section.

Benefits

As an Occupational Therapy student at the University of New Mexico, I would often comment that I hoped to combine my yoga training with an Occupational Therapy approach. While working in the school system and studying Sensory Integration, I began comparing the benefits achieved through yoga with the results of conventional S.I. treatment. It quickly became apparent to me that yoga and S.I. techniques facilitate many of the same functional outcomes for children. Table 1 provides a list of the beneficial results obtained by using either yoga or traditional Sensory Integration techniques, supporting my thesis that yoga itself is a form of Sensory Integration.

Table 1: Shared Benefits of Yoga and SI treatment

Increased ability to attend, participate and learn
Increased independence in functional activities
Improved social skills and positive interactions
Decreased anxiety and fear / less stress
Spontaneous expression of new skills & abilities
Improved motor planning for fine motor skills
Enhanced communication: Listening skills and expressing needs
Ability to handle distractions/interruptions
Increased ability to adjust to changes (flexibility!)
More experiences of joy and fun
Improved ability to regulate own level of alertness
Increased self-esteem, confidence & motivation

Guiding Principles of SI

Simultaneous stimulation of multiple sensory channels is a basic standard of Sensory Integration treatment. Often, we will see a child who is just overwhelmed with all the competing forms of sensory information coming into the brain from the environment. In a chaotic situation, it may be very difficult to know which incoming information is important and which of it can be filtered out. In order to help facilitate that filtering process for children, we as therapists can provide a more structured approach where multiple systems are all stimulated together for the same purposeful activity. This helps the child learn how to integrate multiple sensory systems and decrease those experiences of being overwhelmed by all the sensory stimulation that surrounds us all day.

As previously mentioned, Sensory Integration is based upon the foundation of modulating primarily the tactile, proprioceptive and vestibular systems. In treating the whole child, Sensory Integration also involves two other very powerful sense operations: the visual system and the auditory system. For children to process auditory information accurately and efficiently, it is helpful for three or more sensory channels to be stimulated simultaneously. "Sit still and listen" is nearly impossible for some children because they need a combination of sensory experiences for the auditory system to function optimally. Table 2 shows how the SMILY approach provides stimulation of multiple sensory channels, effectively supporting the development of auditory processing skills.

Table 2: Multiple Sensory Channels

SYSTEM	SMILY INPUT
Tactile: Sense of touch	Encourage removal of socks and shoes for tactile input to bare feet. Feel of mat or floor under palms of hands in certain poses. Finger painting activities.
Proprioception: Muscle and joint sensations; body awareness in space	Weight bearing through various joints of the body, especially in balancing poses and on hands. Repetitive flow of each routine increases awareness of changing body positions through a predictable sequence of postures.
Vestibular System: Balance, muscle tone, motor control, postural control, auditory language skills, attention	Each posture and transition movements between them bring the head in and out of every angle and position relative to the body, with changing directions and speed. Yoga provides alternating stop/start motions, as well as alternating flexion and extension poses.
Visual System: **Visual motor** skills refer to the actions of the tiny muscles that move the eyes, as well the ability of the hand to translate what the eyes see onto paper (copying). **Visual processing** skills refer to discrimination, visual memory, sequencing, closure, etc.	Use of stick figures for imitation of posture, sequencing skills, spatial relations, visual memory and visual discrimination (determining differences between postures). SMILY activities involving tracing, cutting, copying, matching and sequencing skills.
Auditory: Processing of heard information, discrimination between sounds, sound recognition & production.	Story telling with discussion; repetitive singing with rhyming lyrics, paired with vestibular input very powerful!

In order for a session to truly follow the sensory integrative model, it must follow a number of fundamental precepts. A review of the S.I. literature reveals 8 basic principles underlying any Sensory Integration treatment session. Table 3 shows how the SMILY program meets these requirements.

Table 3: Principles of Sensory Integrative Treatment

PRINCIPLE	SMILY APPROACH
Aimed at brainstem and subcortical areas (less cortical activity)	Yoga, breathing and relaxation quiet the cortex, allowing lower brain levels to function more freely, and balance the autonomic nervous system
Strong sensory system strengthens and compensates for weaker systems	Consistently provides input through multiple sensory channels
Helps to regulate the central nervous system's state of alertness	By providing start/stop motions and alternating flexion and extension movements, gives input to vestibular system. Breathing acts as an equalizer to either calm or energize as needed.
Can increase ability for midline activities	Poses alternate rhythmic crossing of midline with maintaining midline orientation; singing induces oral motor focus at midline; fine motor activities
Should be purposeful, goal directed and precede a functional task, known as the "adaptive response"	Movement, singing and relaxation followed by functional fine motor and visual motor activities to improve literacy skills
Activity demands need to be graded	Therapist can increase or decrease sensory input. Child can be allowed to watch, just sing, or just move and gradually combine the skills
Should be FUN for the child	The children say so themselves!
The new behavior must be repeated to become part of child's repertoire	Each session repeats all parts of SMILY many times until motor planning becomes automatic motor memory

Adaptive Responses

The overall desired outcome of sensory integrative treatment is known as the adaptive response. In the words of Dr. Ayres:

> An adaptive response is a purposeful, goal-directed response to a sensory experience...In an adaptive response, we master a challenge and learn something new. At the same time, the formation of an adaptive response helps the brain to develop and organize itself... Play consists of the adaptive responses that make sensory integration happen. The child who learns to organize his play is more likely to organize his school work and become an organized adult.

Adaptive responses occur throughout each SMILY session. Self-initiated modifications and learning can be seen in the children during any phase: breathing, singing, postures, relaxation, and fine motor activities. Adaptive responses can also be more behavioral in context, relating to social interactions and participation levels. Table 4 provides examples of adaptive responses as they relate to education and shows how the SMILY program facilitates them.

Table 4: Adaptive responses facilitated by SMILY

TYPE OF RESPONSE	EXAMPLE	SMILY APPROACH
Attention Skills	Decreased distractibility Focused visual attention	Breathing brings focus Practice of relaxation Visual gaze for balance
Organizational Skills; Following Directions; Task Completion	Gather materials Maintain work space	Auditory processing stimulated by multi-sensory input; children responsible for mats, coming to table
Play and peer relationships/ Group interactions	Turn taking Share area and materials	Take turns practicing sequence, song, sounds Sharing materials
Learning and work skills	Observe skills of others Work alone	Small group activity Encourage completion

The treatment goal is to facilitate adaptive responses that constitute the "just-right challenge" for each child. The SMILY approach is to modify activity demands so that the student is challenged to improve performance but is not distressed through the effort. For example, assistance may be necessary for motor planning either the postures or the fine motor activity. A student may need help organizing his drawings into the correct sequence when creating the book. Opportunities to adjust the challenge are numerous.

Generalization

Generalization is a vital element of learning. It means that a child can take information from one experience and translate it to another time and place. As teachers and therapists, we want our students to be able to generalize what they learn in our lessons to other environments. This means that the specific skills gained in the classroom or during therapy carry over into the rest of the child's life. Learning about safety at school through the practice of fire drills is a good example. Children can apply their knowledge of how to respond in case of fire at home or any other building. Another example is the use of pictures to teach children how to read Exit signs or Stop signs. They are then able to understand the meaning of these signs in the community and put them to functional use. With regard to the SMILY program, I talk with my students about using deep breathing at other times in their lives, such as before a test or when going to sleep at night. Regular practice of relaxation during a yoga session helps children learn how to relax under more stressful circumstances, which often are unpredictable. The movement skills gained through participation in SMILY can increase confidence on the playground and in P.E. It is through generalization of specific skills that children increase their options for interacting with the environment and developing greater self-esteem.

The ability to generalize emerges automatically from a centrally programmed pattern; no cortical planning is needed, just refinement. Experts in the field of sensory-motor development have shown that the paired practice of **imitation** and **sequencing** are essential for motor planning skills. As new, non-habitual activities become familiar and more automatic, motor planning skills transform into sensory-motor memory. It is this sensory-motor memory that supports the ability to generalize because it occurs at a sub-cortical level. As we have shown, the SMILY program operates at the sub-cortical level. SMILY is therefore a valuable tool for enhancing generalization skills through repetition, imitation and sequencing in a multi-sensory environment. It is a therapeutic process that carries over into the classroom to improve behavior and performance.

SECTION THREE:
Research and Literature Review

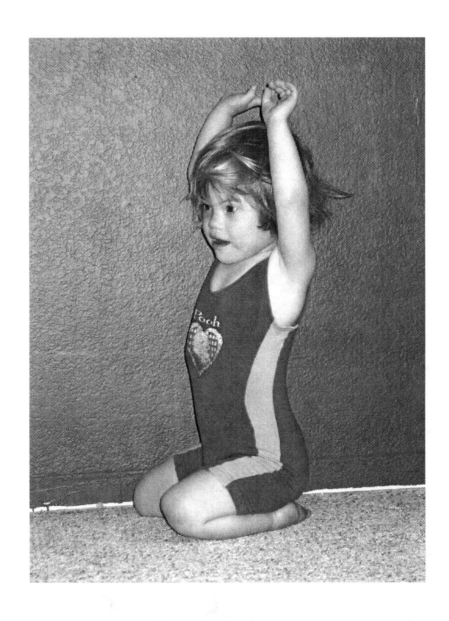

We all are aware of the importance of linking our services with evidence based methods. In this day of limited resources and time constraints, it is important that we avail ourselves of the research and literature that support the therapeutic modalities we include in our treatment planning. The use of programs such as SMILY for educational purposes is well supported by the researchers and authors investigating the important components of childhood development. SMILY as a complete approach combines the principles of music and movement with brain development and literacy skill building.

Previously, are tables listing the noticeable benefits of yoga and Sensory Integrative techniques. Here is evidence based justification for using SMILY as an effective means of helping children learn and succeed in the educational environment. Published sources researching music, movement, yoga, childhood development, learning and literacy overlap widely. Consider for yourself how the creative combination of all these areas, as found in the SMILY program, could be maximally beneficial to the children we teach and serve.

Table 5 provides the details of six different research studies performed over the last several years to determine the efficacy of using yoga to enhance motor skills, cognitive abilities, social adaptation and relaxation. I have included the details here as an overview. Please refer to the "Reference" section at the back of this book if you would like to read the full articles. For now, discover that virtually any level of yoga training with children brings remarkable improvements in mental, physical and emotional foundations.

Table 5: Research on Yoga for Children

SOURCE	METHOD	FINDINGS
Sonia Sumar and Renata Sumar, Yoga for the Special Child (1998)	8 children ages 3-14 years all with Down's Syndrome. Received 2 half hour sessions weekly for 2-3 years. Compared with two control groups who did not do yoga: one with Down's and one without any disabilities	3 areas tested: gross motor, communication and personal/social. Scores in yoga group **higher in every area** than other group with Down's and **very close to scores** of children without disabilities.
Sonia Sumar and Renata Sumar, Yoga for the Special Child (1998)	One 9 year old boy with Cerebral Palsy did yoga 3 times a week for 4 months as adjuct to regular weekly PT & OT	Benefits: quieting of nervous system; better use of arms; focusing attention; improved breathing patterns; greater self-regulation; higher self-esteem
K.V. Naveen, et al, Psychological Reports, volume 81 (1997)	135 children ages 10-17 divided into yoga group and control group. Yoga group practiced specific breathing exercises daily for 10 days.	Testing of perceptual skills involved in memory and spatial relations. All yoga breathing improved spatial memory scores over the control group.
K. Uma, et al, Journal of Mental Deficiency, volume 33 (1989)	90 children with mild, moderate or severe mental retardation, ages 6-15, divided into yoga group and control group. Lessons 5 times a week (one hour) for one year.	Testing of IQ levels and social maturity resulted in those with mild to mod retardation having "highly significant improvement" in all areas.
S. Telles, et al, Perceptual and Motor Skills, volume 81 (1997)	40 girls ages 12-16 divided into yoga group and control group. Yoga practiced one hour daily for 6 months.	Tests measuring symptoms of stress indicate much lower heart rates, slowed respiratory rates and more rhythmic breathing patterns.
S. Telles, et al, Perceptual and Motor Skills, volume 76 (1993)	90 children ages 9-13 divided into yoga group and control group. Intensive yoga lessons daily for 10 days.	Measurements of hand steadiness show that yoga improves motor control, coordination and concentration.

Observational Outcomes of Yoga for Children

I have been teaching yoga to children for over five years, and have been so thrilled to see the progress they make through on-going practice. Many of the children I am working with have been with me for three years or more. I can say that yoga training is not a "quick fix"; it does take time, practice and repetition. In the beginning it may even seem like the challenge is too great; you may think that the postures or the sequencing is too difficult for some children. But stick with it – you will see positive gains before too long. And, be sure to read the "How to Teach Children" section for specific tips on how to assist or modify poses.

Within the first year with many of my students, I started to see exciting improvements. I will never forget the experience of working with a 9 year old boy with Attention Deficit Hyperactivity Disorder. Let's call him Luke. Even with his medication, Luke had a very difficult time focusing his attention or keeping his body still for any significant length of time. He was virtually unable to stay on his yoga mat. This went on for a few months, with Luke being present in the room while the rest of the small group of 9 year old boys participated fully in the program. Yes, there were times when his behavior was distracting and Luke needed to take some time away from the group, for everybody's benefit. He wanted to be there though, and made efforts to stay with the other boys, who pointedly asked him to try doing the yoga with them. After a while, he began to take an interest in learning the belly breathing technique. Then he started to participate in the "Dreamer" section of each class. In less than one school year, Luke was able to perform very nice, deep belly breathing without any instruction or cueing from me at all. And, he could lie perfectly still in relaxation for at least 3 minutes, without any signs of distractibility! That was one of the most rewarding outcomes I have experienced yet.

In addition to helping with attention and concentration, I have also witnessed steady improvement in children's ability to perform yoga postures. With repetition, practice and support, yoga training can and does improve strength, balance, flexibility and coordination. I have seen children unable to move smoothly from one posture to the next, collapsing on the floor and very often seeming to just give up. But, we all keep trying. And over time, these students develop an ability to sequence the series of postures with much better timing, coordination and endurance. In particular, I have watched children progress from a complete inability to stand on one leg to holding a balancing posture for 5 or even 10 seconds without wavering! Practice, practice, practice.

Improvement in the physical skills of balance, coordination, strength and stamina are all excellent outcomes in and of themselves. These components alone make yoga a worthy method for us all. With children, especially those who have special needs, the most wonderful aspect to see unfolding is the growth of confidence and self-esteem that occurs as a result of mastering these physical tasks. Many of my students will note their own progress, commenting on poses they once had difficulty doing. They will begin to report which poses they are good at, and are eager to share their new found skills. And, they also tell me that yoga is fun. They enjoy it, it helps them, and they know that.

Movement, Brain Development and Learning

A study of the literature available regarding the role of movement in learning reveals numerous authors and researchers working to solidify the link between moving and thinking. Current brain research points to the direct connection between body and mind, and how physical movement is beneficial for brain function. Of particular interest lately has been the role of one sub-cortical region of the brain known as the **cerebellum**, adjacent to the brain stem at the bottom of the rear brain. For many years, it was believed that the only role of the cerebellum was to regulate motor functions for accuracy, timing, balance and coordination. For example, it is the cerebellum that allows us to reach for a glass of water and bring it to our lips with the exact amount of muscle force and speed needed to take a drink. For these functions, the cerebellum is connected to the major cortical area of the brain known as the motor cortex. Previously, it was thought that this was the only significant connection of the cerebellum with the rest of the brain.

More recent studies have shown that the cerebellum is also linked with many other sub-cortical regions of the brain believed to play a significant role in thinking and learning. For example, it has been found by neurologists that patients with cerebellar damage also show impaired cognitive abilities along with coordination and balance deficits – thereby linking movement and thinking at a functional level. In addition, cerebellar dysfunction has also been linked with an impaired ability to shift attention from one activity to another in a smooth, efficient manner. It is now believed that the cerebellum coordinates not only accurate motor skills, but also paves the way for decision making processes by modulating many levels of motor and sensory based information (including emotional responses). The cerebellum is now considered to play a primary role as the "relay station" for cognitive functions.

Eric Jensen, author of numerous books including <u>Teaching with the Brain in Mind</u> and <u>The Learning Brain</u>, refers to hands-on learning (like riding a bike) as "intrinsic learning" that occurs through physical experiences. Explicit learning, (like hearing the state capitols) may be quicker, but learning through physical action creates more neural networks in the brain. Jensen strongly supports movement as an important way of enriching brain function. He writes that enrichment results in:

- Heavier nerve cells in the Central Nervous System (CNS)
- More glial cells (foundational cellular elements of the CNS)
- Greater dendritic branching (more projections of nerve cell fibers)
- Multiple synaptic junctions (contact of one nerve cell with another)

Due to this resulting increase in neural connections, Jensen says, motor skills are fundamental to learning and memory is better retrieved through movement.

It is important to make a distinction between two related brain functions that link movement with learning. The skill known as **motor planning** refers to the ability to carry out unfamiliar or novel actions in a skilled manner. This function occurs within cortical regions of the brain known as the motor cortex. The frontal lobe in particular helps us with the problem solving, sequencing and decision making involved in performing new actions (as when we first learn how to drive). Over time, novel movements become familiar and are stored as **motor memory.** Motor memory skills involve precise recall of learned patterns for consistent, automatic movements (as seen with experienced drivers, dancers, athletes, etc.). The SMILY program enhances this connection between motor planning and motor memory: when we begin a new routine, children are working at the level of motor planning as they learn the new movements. With repetition, the routine becomes familiar and is performed using motor memory skills. Motor memory functions are performed at sub-cortical levels of the cerebellum and other related brain regions. Table 6 provides a list of some primary areas of the brain that are either directly connected to the cerebellum or help to perform related functions important to thinking and learning.

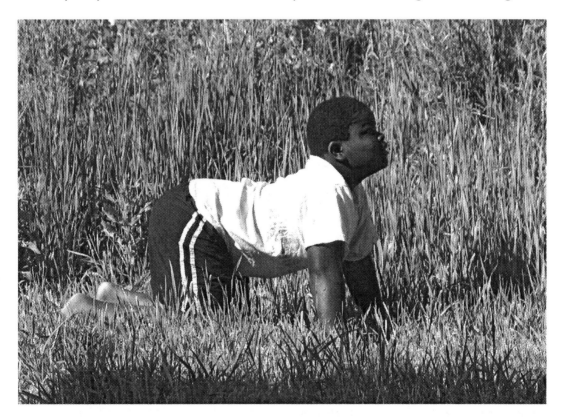

Table 6: Learning in the Brain

BRAIN REGION	FUNCTION
Cerebrum/Cerebral Cortex/ Hemispheres: Outer layer of brain structures. Each side of the brain has frontal, parietal, temporal and occipital lobes and specific cortical areas known as motor cortex and sensory cortex.	Higher brain functions of sensation, voluntary muscle movement, thought, reasoning and memory. Frontal lobes involved in decision making, planning, problem solving, impulse control. Temporal lobes involved in language processing and categorization of sound.
Corpus Callosum: large structure of nerve fibers just below the cerebral cortex, connecting the right and left hemispheres	Most communication between different regions in the two sides of the brain carried over by the corpus callosum – a "freeway" between cortical areas.
Basal Ganglia: groups of nerve cell bodies deep in the brain closely associated with cerebellum and motor cortex	Receive inputs from motor areas and send projections back to cerebral cortex to modify movements; fine tuning of voluntary or willed movements
Vestibular Nuclei: nerve cell bodies located in the brainstem; together with inner ear structures and the Vestibular Nerve (Cranial Nerve VIII) they comprise the Vestibular System. Vestibular Nuclei closely modulated by cerebellum.	Mediation of electrical signaling within the Vestibular System. Receive signals related to head movement from the Vestibular Nerve and project impulses to Oculomotor Nuclei which drive eye muscle activity
Reticular Activating System (RAS): a fine network of nerve cells near top of brain-stem activated by the Vestibular Nuclei	Regulates incoming sensory data to help turn thinking into action and to govern attention, concentration and pleasure.

Having familiarized ourselves with the primary functions of specific brain regions needed for learning, we can now turn to the question of brain development. How can we help support the acquisition and growth of these functions in children? Experts in the field of brain research are some of the strongest proponents of providing a variety of movement experiences to stimulate brain development early in life. Table 7 reviews the work of several authors, indicating that the use of programs such as SMILY can greatly enhance learning.

Table 7: Theories of Brain Development

SOURCE	STATEMENTS/CONCLUSIONS
Shatz, C., "The Developing Brain", Scientific American vol 267:3 (1992)	We do not add brain cells as we grow older, but do lose them through the aging process. The number of brain cells is not nearly as important as the **number of interconnections between them.**
Shore, R., Rethinking the Brain: New Insights into Early Development (1997)	If we don't use neural connections often enough, the brain "disengages" them. A wide variety of repetitive activities are essential to early brain development.
Jensen, E., Teaching with the Brain in Mind (1998)	Movement helps to lay down the neural pathways that strengthen memory and learning. Exercise makes the corpus callosum, basal ganglia and cerebellum stronger.
Sylwester, R., A Biological Brain in a Cultural Classroom: Enhancing Cognitive and Social Development through Collaborative Classroom Management (2001)	A central mission of the brain is to intelligently navigate its environment. Since efficient movement facilitates cognition, the curriculum must include movement concepts and skills.
Ratey, J., A User's Guide to the Brain: Perception, Attention and the Four Theaters of the Brain (2001)	Our physical movements can directly influence our ability to learn, think, and remember...Evidence is mounting that each person's capacity to master new and remember old information is improved by biological changes brought on by physical activity. Our physical movements call upon some of the same neurons used for reading, writing, and math...What makes us move also makes us think.
Gardner, H., Frames of Mind: The Theory of Multiple Intelligences (1992 tenth edition)	**Bodily-Kinesthetic Intelligence** is a primary means of learning: The individual's perception of the world is itself affected by the status of his motor activities. Information concerning the position and status of the body itself regulates the way in which subsequent perception of the world takes place...In the absence of such feedback from motor activity, perception cannot develop in a normal way.

April Merrilee

Music and Childhood Development

One childhood experience for which I am so very grateful was the opportunity to participate in music lessons, including piano and clarinet, from a young age until my teen years. Fortunately, I have recently returned to playing piano after 20 years without any practice at all. It brings me so much pleasure to sit down and play. More to the point is this: I am absolutely amazed at the ability of the brain to remember a motor activity after so many years, retrieve it, and process it into the output of a song! From my own personal experience, I firmly believe that the musical training I received was a very important component of my own development – not only for motor control but also the fundamental cognitive skills of attention, memory, sequencing, and problem solving. I believe my early musical experiences supported my growth as a student and helped me to learn from a wide variety of educational environments.

While researching sources for this section, I came across the work of Lili M. Levinowitz – music education professor at Rowan University of New Jersey. I was particularly impressed with her article, **"The Importance of Music in Early Childhood"**, published in <u>General Music Today</u> by the Music Educators National Conference, Fall 1998. She paints a very clear picture of music as a developmental skill in its own right. Levinowitz makes these very important points with regard to the need for musical training in the lives of children:

- Making music is as much a basic life skill as walking or talking.
- Even the youngest infant is wired to receive music.
- Music research indicates that, like language development, young children develop musically through a predictable sequence to basic music competence, which includes **singing in tune and marching to a beat.**
- The most typical negative influence on developmental music aptitude is simply neglect...Without sufficient stimulation and exposure, the inborn potential for musical growth may actually atrophy.

Perhaps most relevant to a consideration of SMILY as a means of providing musical experiences to children is Levinowitz's discussion of the process involved in gaining the ability to perform music accurately. This unfolding occurs as the result of two developmental components:

    1) <u>**Kinesthetic awareness**</u>: through the actions of singing and moving, the body itself is used as a type of musical instrument for a kinesthetic experience of music.

    2) <u>**Audiation**</u>: the complex mental process of "unscrambling" the images of music; how the brain learns to receive, register and process categories of sound. (The Sensory Integrative description of music!)

Levinowitz concludes with some of the best professional support for participating in the SMILY program I have found:

"From a developmental perspective, children must experience rhythm **in their bodies** before they can successfully audiate in their minds. The early childhood years are crucial for using the body to respond as a musical instrument **in many ways to many different kinds of music**."

Research on Music and Childhood Development

Table 8 summarizes recent findings of educators, music researchers and childhood development specialists regarding the benefits of providing musical stimulation to children. From a vast array of support for the use of music in education, here is a relevant sampling of the available literature.

Table 8: Music and Childhood Development

SOURCE	CONCLUSIONS
Cassidy, J and Standley J, "The Effect of Music Listening on Physiological Responses of Premature Infants in the NICU", Journal of Music Therapy vol 32 (1995)	Of 20 infants with gestation times of 24-30 weeks, 10 listened to lullabies at timed intervals. Compared to control group, the music group had "noticeably positive effects on oxygen saturation levels, heart rate and respiratory rate."
Mitchell, D. "The Relationship between Rhythmic Competency and Academic Performance", University of Central Florida (2003)	Young children with developed rhythm skills perform better academically in early school years. High scores on rhythmic tasks link with high academic achievement as compared to lower rhythmic scores.
Schlag, Gottfried, et al, Nature (1995)	Musicians have larger corpus callosum, motor cortex and left temporal lobe.
Buday, "The Effects of Signed and Spoken Words Taught with Music on Sign and Speech Imitation by Children with Autism", Journal of Music Therapy, vol 32 (1995)	Study of 10 children with autism receiving music and rhythm lessons along with speech and sign language. Showed significant effects from music training, with greater correct imitation of both signed words and spoken words.
Rauscher, et al, "Music training causes long term enhancement of preschool children's spatial-temporal reasoning", Neurological Research, vol 19 (1997)	Compared 78 children receiving either music or computer lessons with control group. Only the music group showed significant improvement on tests of spatial reasoning, showing possible causal link.
Palmer, H., "The Music, Movement and Learning Connection", Young Child (Sept. 2001)	Music and movement combinations are especially beneficial to learning because they engage the whole child with active involvement in repetition, rhythm, rhyme and alliteration.

Supporting Literacy Skills

The first assumption when we hear the word "literacy" is to think of teaching people how to read. Remember that the broader view of literacy refers to someone who can both **read and write**. Further in this text, I detail the functional components of reading and handwriting skills and show how the SMILY approach addresses them. Here is a sampling of the relevant literature supporting the use of a program such as SMILY to enhance the development of literacy skills. Table 9 summarizes the statements I've gathered from a variety of experts in the field of education, particularly in the areas of language development and literacy.

Table 9: Literacy Skill Building

SOURCE	STATEMENTS/CONCLUSIONS
Neuman, Copple and Bredekamp, Learning to Read and Write: Developmentally Appropriate Practices for Young Children (2000)	Rhymes, rhythms and repetition sensitize children to the sounds of language, or phonemes. Phonemic awareness is an important predictor of later success in reading.
Balzer-Martin, L. Sensory Integration: Theory, Assessment, Treatment and Screening Program for Young Children, a MEDS-PDN seminar publication (2003)	Phonemic awareness is a bilateral function of the brain performed via the corpus callosum linking two components of reading: sound recognition (right brain) and sound production (left brain)
Asher, J.J., Learning Another Language through Activities: The Complete Teacher's Guide (1996)	Understanding word meaning is the first step in developing oral and written communication skills... understanding is enhanced through movement...there is a direct relationship between language and the body.

Table 9 continued

Block, B.A., "Literacy through Movement: An Organized Approach", <u>Journal of Physical Education, Recreation and Dance</u>, vol 72 (2001)	Children should listen to the rhythm of language and actively participate in **physical expressions of this rhythm**...this teaches them to be aware of the rhythm of literary works and to internalize the beat.
Pica, R., <u>Linking Literacy and Movement</u> & <u>Moving and Learning Across the Curriculum</u> (1999)	Linking words to form sentences (and eventually paragraphs) is very similar to stringing movements together to form sequences...Both require that children choose components that naturally flow... Both require breathing room (a pause) and an ending (period).
Hannaford, C., <u>Smart Moves: Why Learning is Not All in Your Head</u> (1995)	We have spent years and resources struggling to teach people to learn, and yet the standardized test scores go down and illiteracy rises. Could it be that one of the key elements we've been missing is simply movement?

SECTION FOUR:

Components of Learning and the SMILY Approach

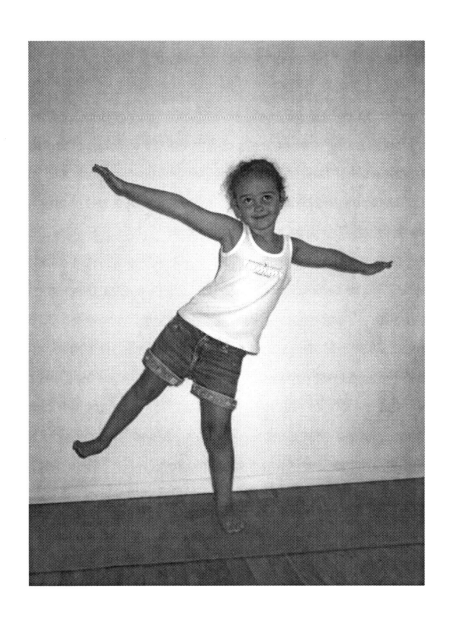

Sensory Motor Components of Learning

Now let's consider how the concepts of sensory integration relate to classroom performance. In many children with special needs, the sensory-motor system is often dysfunctional. This dysfunction can occur at any level of this "feedback" loop:
- Stimulation of sensory-motor receptors
- Registering the information in the brain
- Processing all the various sensory motor input
- Formulating a behavioral or motor response
- Performing the desired behavior or motor output

Sensory Integration treatment seeks to optimize all portions of this sensory-motor processing loop in order to enhance a child's ability to focus attention, learn, and produce classroom work. Table 10 outlines the primary sensory and motor components related to learning and behavior, and shows how the SMILY program enhances these requisite abilities for classroom performance.

All of these components in combination come into play as a child explores the environment and "learns how to learn". Experts tell us that processing information – particularly auditory input– is best accomplished when provided through multiple sensory channels. The SMILY program greatly emphasizes the combination of vestibular, proprioceptive and auditory systems in every session. I feel this multi-sensory approach is of great benefit to children. When a child is having difficulty with classroom performance, these components should be taken into consideration. Please refer to Table 10 to review the sensory motor components of learning.

Table 10: Sensory and Motor Components of Learning

COMPONENT	FUNCTION	SMILY APPROACH
Auditory Processing	Ability to understand what is heard, associate sounds with meaning, follow directions	Simultaneous stimulation of several sensory channels; use of music and movement
Body Awareness	Knowing where body is and how it is moving in space without vision	Graded input using verbal directions and hands-on help; verbal feedback
Coordinating Body Sides	Core stability; using both sides of brain; crossing midline; front/back, right/left, top/bottom and rotational movements	Postures alternate midline orientation and crossing; spatial concepts taught through visual and kinesthetic input
Motor Planning	Conceive of, organize and carry out skilled, unfamiliar actions	Each routine initially unfamiliar; emphasis on sequencing important
Motor Memory	Recall patterns for consistent, automatic movements	Repetitious practice of same sequence; visual aid of stick figures
Fine Motor Control	Use of hands and fingers in skilled activity	Poses build upper body strength and enhance eye-hand coordination
Ocular Control	Smooth movements of eyes for finding moving object, keeping eye contact on fixed object and eye-hand coordination	Present stick figures in left to right sequence; demo poses in flow fashion; use of visual gaze for balance
Visual-Spatial Perception and Processing	Perceiving the relationship between objects in space	Use yoga mat as personal boundary; start/stop stimulation of vestibular system; copying activities

Table 10 continued

Visual Discrimination	Distinguishing similar and different shapes and letters	Pairing printed words with movement; tracing stick figures; visual memory games
Perception of Movement	Processing vestibular information to help maintain posture, balance and motor control	All yoga postures provide combination of vestibular and proprioceptive input; breathing and sequencing
Perception of Touch or Tactile Input	Sense of touch on the skin (light or deep)	Hands-on assistance; deep pressure for relaxation; varied tactile input during fine motor; strongly encourage bare feet

Handwriting Skills

I support the current view of handwriting as a combination of both **motor** and **language skills**. Language itself is a pre-requisite skill for handwriting. A child needs to understand spatial concepts and the directional words related to them before being able to form letters correctly. Comprehending spatial relations, direction, and left/right discrimination begins with and is sustained by movement. Movement can be initiated through verbal directions using specific spatial terms.

It is best if the child is able to conceive of spatial language both verbally and physically. Thus, the pairing of movement with song is an ideal method for laying down the spatial language concepts inherent to handwriting. Combining body awareness with spatial concepts in a multi-sensory environment nicely complements any handwriting program. This is exactly what the SMILY routines provide.

Fundamental handwriting skills are developed through activities that enhance a child's ability to copy shapes and forms. Copy skills are not limited to figures on paper, but also include imitation of movement sequences and the auditory input of song. Joanne Landy and Keith Burridge elaborate on the role of movement and music in their work, <u>Fine Motor Skills and Handwriting Activities for Young Children</u>. They state that "motor memory relates to the ability to visually and auditorially copy movements, movement patterns and rhythm patterns." As previously shown, motor memory is a central part of the SMILY program that contributes greatly to the development of handwriting skills. Table 11 outlines the specific motor abilities needed for a child to master handwriting.

Table 11: Motor Components of Handwriting

DEFINITION	SMILY APPROACH
Postural Stability: Strength and efficiency of core muscles along spine, pelvis, abdomen; trunk balance for sitting and dynamic movements.	All yoga poses involve the use of deep postural muscles used for static and dynamic balance. Repetition builds core strength; poses become easier with practice and the muscular effort becomes easier and more efficient.
Midline Orientation: Ability to perform focused tasks directly in front of the body, as well as shifting movements away from midline and back again.	Yoga develops the tiny muscles along the spine so that the trunk stays erect during fine motor activities. The sequenced routines develop smooth transitional movements between poses, with focus shifting in and out of midline throughout the session.
Timing and Rhythm: ability to perform refined, accurate movements in a coordinated manner.	Pairing movement with music helps to coordinate the motions of upper and lower body. Clapping in unison with group helps with accuracy and precision.
Visual Motor Integration: ability to smoothly combine motor tasks with eye muscle function, and the processing of visual information	Use of stick figure drawings as point of visual attention during routines, as well as imitation of posture while watching demonstration of poses. Followed by fine motor tasks involving visual perceptual, visual motor and eye-hand coordination tasks.
Bilateral Integration: ability of upper and lower extremities to work together to perform coordinated actions	Imitation of yoga postures teaches the two sides of the body work together efficiently. Fine motor tasks enhance coordination during table top activities.
Grading Muscle Contraction: innate knowledge of precise amount of muscle force needed to perform motor activities.	Yoga practice conditions muscles to work efficiently, without excess tension or effort. Pairing movement with music helps improve awareness of body, position and strength.
Upper Extremity Strength: Includes superficial and deep muscles of upper back and chest; shoulder girdle; arms, hands and fingers.	Many postures use weight bearing on hands to increase shoulder stability, and strength of intrinsic muscles of hand and extrinsic muscles of forearm; upper body function achieved through stimulation of vestibular system.

Naturally, the fine motor activities set up as adaptive responses at the end of each routine provide the practice and repetition needed for handwriting. The opportunity for tracing shapes and letters is particularly helpful for children who struggle with formation or sizing/spacing issues. Vary the tactile options by offering different writing materials, including colored pencils, markers, and crayons.

Upon reviewing many sources dedicated to improving handwriting skills in children, it became apparent that there are 5 distinct models of handwriting intervention. Table 12 shows how the SMILY program uses them all.

Table 12: Handwriting Models of Intervention

MODEL	EXAMPLES	SMILY APPROACH
Biomechanical	Address motor control issues and postural concerns	Imitation of posture, repetition and sequencing to increase motor memory skills for smooth movements
Neuromuscular	Balance and stability in sitting; regulation of muscle tone; shoulder stability	Weight bearing on hands for shoulder stability; regulation of muscle tone through vestibular system; balancing postures
Acquisitional	Skill taught through practice, applied to different contexts, short lessons	Tracing, changing routines and vary fine motor activities (10 minutes at end)
Multi-sensory	SI input, material changes, position changes	Stimulation of multiple sensory channels in preparation for fine motor; various writing implements; seating options
Motivational	Self-esteem, FUN, success, one-on-one	Confidence, grade activity for success

Literacy Skills

One of the most wonderful ways that the SMILY program connects yoga with learning is through language development. This starts from the very first session by displaying the song lyrics as well as the names of the stick figure drawings, and continues into specific activities for each routine. Literacy teachers are skilled at finding ways to raise lifelong readers. Table 13 shares some of the tips I have picked up along the way.

Table 13: Encouraging Literacy

SUGGESTION	SMILY APPROACH
Create reading rituals: designate a quality time to read together; let reading be a way to connect with the children in your life	Each SMILY session can be approached as a reading ritual by consistently including all the aspects of each routine. Given as a coherent program, all the components serve to stimulate literacy skills.
Keep a running conversation about the reading material	Especially during the fine motor activities, talk about the story and its characters. Let the original story spur questions relating to life and learning.
Surround children with words: both spoken and written	Words are central to every SMILY session: printed on all the materials; sung to melodies; used in conversation, etc.
Relate reading and writing to a special interest or hobby	Literacy components are inherent to the context of each routine; the reading and writing activities are directly related to the music and movement framework

Remember that writing supports reading and vice versa. The fine motor activities are all designed to make handwriting more fun and enjoyable, and are directly linked to the story and song of each SMILY routine. This contextual approach provides three key elements that are found in any literacy program:

- **STRUCTURE:** Activities are presented in the same manner for each routine.
- **ORGANIZATION:** Children learn how to use all the different materials.
- **DIRECTION:** Each session follows the same basic format or sequence of events.

Of course, there are fundamental elements that must be included when we aim to facilitate literacy development. Table 14 provides the specific details that are necessary in the effort to teach literacy skills.

Table 14: Components of Literacy Skills

COMPONENTS	SMILY APPROACH
Recognition of Letters (names, shapes) Connect Letter Symbols and Sounds	Printed names of poses by stick figures; lyrics to songs displayed on posterboard. Point to words while singing/speaking.
Expand Vocabulary	Unfamiliar animal names; describe placement of body parts using spatial and directional terms for postures
Story Re-telling	With repetition of routine; Ask children about basic story content , "Who can tell me what happened?"
Comprehension; Higher Order Thinking	Ask children concrete and more abstract questions about story and implications; prediction questions, etc. Discussion of story to enhance literal and reflective understanding.
Exposure to Reading Process	Adult demonstration and child practice pointing at words on posterboard while singing to model the act of reading
Spelling	Visual aides show children patterns of letters and how words are combined. Singing supports fluency. Spells name of poses aloud during routine; children make spelling books and sentence books according to age.
Phonemic Awareness (understanding that spoken words are made up of sequences of sounds)	Greatly enhanced by combination of music and movement stimulating bilateral functions of brain; sequencing of yoga postures; sound repetition while singing
Beginning Writing	Strengthening of upper body and eye-hand coordination. Fine motor activities of tracing, drawing and copying. Visual perceptual skills of discrimination, matching, memory and sequencing.

Multiple Intelligences

In his books, <u>Frames of Mind: The Theory Of Multiple Intelligences</u> and <u>Multiple Intelligences: The Theory into Practice</u>, Howard Gardner suggests that as human beings we all possess different types of learning styles or intelligences. For each of us, certain methods or ways of learning are stronger than others. With regard to childhood development, it is important to offer children a variety of educational formats that speak to all the learning styles. Ideally, as educators we want to generate learning through stimulation of all the different types of intelligence. In this way, we can teach to the whole child rather than focusing on just one or two aspects. Being aware of and acknowledging that different children learn in different ways is an important concept to meeting diverse educational needs. Incorporating a variety of approaches into the curriculum can help broaden the ways in which children are able to learn from their environments.

In addition, by providing diverse experiences we are more likely to accommodate the strongest learning styles within each student. This varied approach thereby allows children to take advantage of their greatest strengths, rather than struggling to compensate and mold themselves into learning styles that don't feel as natural. Instead of clumping different learners into the same category, we can structure activities to offer a greater variety of educational experiences. Table 15 outlines seven different intelligences and how the SMILY program inherently addresses all these learning styles. Isn't it wonderful to know there are functional, educationally relevant ways, to meet the needs of children right where they are?

Table 15: Multiple Intelligences

LEARNING STYLE	SMILY APPROACH
Visual/Spatial Learner: Processes visual information easily and retains through visual memory. Enjoys drawing, painting, spatial relations, building and puzzles.	Presentation of poses through stick figure drawings supports spatial relations; dot-to-dot pictures and visual memory games. Display of lyrics.
Logical/Mathematical Learner: Quick to find patterns, good with numbers and counting. Enjoys solving problems.	Consistent sequencing of poses, paired with song lyrics. Fine motor activities based on correct sequencing of names and drawings. Make up simple math problems while doing activities. Example: If we've drawn 5 of the poses, how many more are left?
Bodily/Kinesthetic Learner: Has good physical coordination and balance skills. Demonstrates strength in fine motor activities. Enjoys lots of movement.	Yoga postures provide the bodily experience that stimulates the sense of kinesthesia. Fine motor activities linked to greater context of gross motor exercises.
Verbal/Linguistic Learner: Skilled at expressing self through words. Likes to create and hear stories and rhymes.	Each routine begins with a story that is carried through the music and movement portion and continued into structured follow-up activities. Lots of rhymes and overall language development!
Interpersonal Learner: Act as leaders in groups, are outgoing and empathetic towards others.	SMILY is always given in a group format, either as a small pull-out group or with the whole class as an inclusion activity. Some children act as great models for the music and movement, and can also model effective work behaviors during fine motor tasks.
Intrapersonal Learner: May appear quiet or inner directed but are very self-confident and at peace with themselves.	Beginning each session with belly breathing and practicing Dreamer for relaxation supports the sense of inner peace. Physical postures and fine motor projects are done independently; success generates even more self-confidence.
Musical/Rhythmic Learner: Loves to create and listen to music. Often hum, sing and keep time to music from an early age.	SMILY is singing! We also clap, and move our bodies to the rhythm of the song. Many children continue to hum or sing while we do the fine motor activities.

SECTION FIVE:
In the School Setting

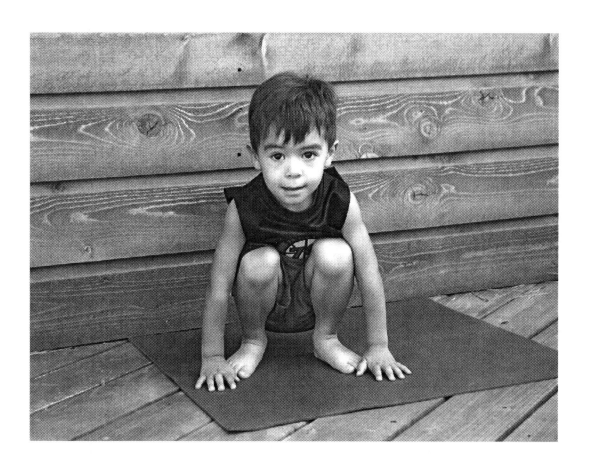

42

Multi-Disciplinary Approach

As an experienced school based therapist, I am committed to the value of the co-treatment approach. Simultaneous treatment sessions for any combination of Occupational, Physical and Speech Therapists, as well as Resource Teachers, are beneficial in a number of ways. Logistically, it can often be quite complicated and indeed difficult to find convenient times within a student's school day to provide therapy. Combining therapies into overlapping sessions leaves more time for the student with special needs to stay involved with the regular education class. I believe it is particularly important that all students participate in library, computer, physical education, and fine arts with their class as much as possible. Those times are not readily available for therapy, and this is also obviously true of lunch and recess times too. Therapists and teachers frequently find ourselves needing to see the same children at the same time; co-treating can be a very valuable solution to the scheduling issue.

Going beyond the sheer practicalities of schedule, a multi-disciplinary approach also involves a shared responsibility to address the specific goals that lend structure to each child's Individualized Education Plan (IEP). For example, as an Occupational Therapist, my goals may focus on increasing bilateral coordination or specific fine motor skills. However, I am also aware of the student's Physical Therapy goals such as increasing balance and strength, or Speech goals targeting specific articulation or fluency concerns. As a team working together, we are better able to support ways in which all disciplines can address their goals within any one session. This means the student is receiving more applicable input within a therapy session where two or more therapists are involved at the same time, consciously addressing a variety of educationally related goals.

A SMILY session can be provided to children in a variety of formats. It works quite well for the familiar method of bringing children out of class for a therapy session. In this case a small group of three or four is ideal for a detailed focus on specific IEP objectives. However, the SMILY program is also easily adapted as an inclusion activity so that direct therapy services can be provided in the regular education setting with the entire class participating. This supports Least Restrictive Environment (LRE) considerations, as students are able to receive therapeutic input without coming away from the regular education class. And, it is a nice opportunity for therapists to co-treat since it is very helpful to have more than one therapist helping to organize the class and maintain a therapeutic quality throughout the activity.

Inclusion based therapy is a "win-win" situation for all involved. Children with special needs enjoy participating with the entire class; they enjoy sharing what they know with others. One very effective method for ensuring their success is to use the SMILY program twice per week: once in a small group format (pull out) and a second time with the regular education class. I particularly like this approach for children with special needs because the first session allows more individualized instruction so that greater learning takes place. With this comes more confidence, so that the student feels prepared for the session in the general classroom. Often the student on my caseload can take a leadership role by helping to teach classmates how to do the routine or its associated lessons. This in turns helps to build more confidence, self-esteem and motivation for continued learning.

As therapists and special educators, our focus is primarily with the children on our caseload. However, it is also worthy to note that a SMILY practice is also of great benefit to all children, whether or not they have special challenges. Many children involved in the SMILY program have expressed their enjoyment of the routines. They tell me how much fun they are having, and often comment on how they are getting better at doing the yoga poses. Sometimes it is fun to experiment with an option referred to as "reverse inclusion". With permission, try occasionally grouping the children on your caseload with just a few students from their regular education classrooms for a special type of pull-out session. This really makes your students feel very important, and helps them forge relationships with classmates.

Optimal sensory-motor development is central to enhancing a child's educational experience. Therefore, all children can benefit from the SMILY program. Furthermore, the classroom teachers who welcome SMILY into their rooms have repeatedly commented on the resulting positive behaviors.

Least Restrictive Environment

Current trends are moving once again toward increasing use of an inclusion based model for service delivery in the Least Restrictive Environment (LRE). SMILY is very well adapted for use as an inclusion activity in both the pre-school and elementary school settings. Table 18 shows how the SMILY program supports the concept of meeting special needs while following the guidelines of providing therapy within the LRE.

Table 16: Least Restrictive Environment

The SMILY program is fully accessible through the general education curriculum, as an inclusion based activity.
Children of varying abilities can participate together without the need to separate those with special needs. SMILY supports the goal of increasing each child's participation in regular classes and school activities.
Those children who truly do require a pull-out session due to special needs can receive a small group format at least once per week as needed.
Use of SMILY allows students with special needs to participate within the regular education setting while also utilizing supplementary aides and services.
The SMILY program inherently follows all necessary conditions set forth in a student's IEP. (See "In the School Setting for IEP's)
The wide reaching components, benefits and benchmarks related to SMILY make it a highly appropriate method of meeting the highly individualized needs of pre-school and elementary age children.
SMILY offers delivery of services in a wide range of placement options, along a continuum ranging from individual, to small group and inclusion. Placement for a student with special needs is only as restrictive as his abilities require.

Very often, one of the first questions I hear from teachers is how to fit the SMILY program into their burgeoning curriculum. At first glance, SMILY feels like another activity to squeeze into an already full schedule. However, benefits can be achieved in as little as 30 minutes per week. Plus, the qualities of improved concentration and enhanced learning can actually serve to save time over the long run as children become more focused and efficient.

One creative idea a group of teachers expressed was to do the music and movement portion as part of a P.E. class, followed by the activities as a Language Arts lesson back in the classroom. How can a SMILY activity qualify as a curriculum based educational lesson? Let's take a look at state educational benchmarks.

General Education Benchmarks

Administrators and teachers are constantly called upon to make good decisions about how to structure classroom time. With the current emphasis on testing under the "No Child Left Behind" policy, it is vital that our students are learning fundamental academic skills. Obviously, time is a valuable resource and we must be sure that we are making good use of it. I am stating in no uncertain terms that SMILY can and does support the basic educational goals we are setting for the children we teach. And how wonderful that it also happens to be so much fun, and brings so many benefits to our students!

As I began developing the SMILY program, I saw that its components were inherently meeting basic educational objectives. I knew right away that by emphasizing language development, SMILY activities would definitely meet instruction requirements in the area of Language Arts. Then I realized how often we are using math concepts: counting, using ordinals, sequencing, drawing shapes, describing spatial relationships. Over time it became more and more apparent to me how thoroughly relevant the SMILY approach is to the general curriculum.

A review of standards from the New Mexico State Board of Education confirms that participation in the SMILY program meets the requirements set forth in the Educational Benchmarks for elementary students (K-4). The academic areas most readily addressed include Language Arts, Mathematics, Physical Education, and Arts Performance. Tables 17-20 give some specific examples from the many that are applicable. Share the following pages with administrators and teachers to boost support for the use of SMILY in your school!

Table 17: Language Arts Benchmarks

STANDARD	BENCHMARK = SMILY APPROACH
Apply strategies and skills to comprehend information that is read, heard, and viewed.	1. Listen to, read, react to, and retell information. 2. Demonstrate familiarity with a variety of resources: pictures; captions; rhymes; stories; plays 3. Demonstrate critical thinking skills to comprehend written, spoken, and visual information: formulate questions about stories; sequence the parts; discuss similarities and differences of characters 4. Acquire reading strategies: phonemic awareness; ecognize letters and their sounds; increase vocabulary
Apply grammatical and language conventions to communicate.	1. Use pictures and context to make predictions about story content 2. Recognize and make complete, coherent sentences when speaking 3. Ask and answer questing about essential elements
Communicate effectively through speaking and writing	1. Use correct words to name objects or tell actions 2. Use a variety of sentence patterns 3. Develop spelling strategies and skills
Use literature and media to develop an understanding of people, societies and the self.	1. Listen and respond to stories based on themes 2. Examine and identify reasons for characters' actions 3. Consider a situation or problem from different characters' point of view. 4. Take part in creative responses to dramatizations, stories and plays. 5. Identify the use of rhythm, rhyme and alliteration
Demonstrate competence in the skills and strategies of the writing process	1. Write all the letters of the alphabet correctly 2. Write own names and names of others 3. Compose a variety of written products (drawing, tracing, copying)

Table 18: Mathematics Benchmarks

STANDARD	BENCHMARK = SMILY APROACH
Understand numbers, ways of representing numbers, relationships among numbers, and number systems.	1. Count with understanding (how many poses are there; counting while in balancing postures) 2. Order sets of objects (sequence pictures) 3. Count orally by 2's, 5's, 10's (while balancing) 4. Use ordinal numbers (while putting pictures in order, name 1st, 2nd, 3rd, 4th, etc.)
Understand geometric concepts and applications	1. Describe, identify, model and draw geometric conceptsobjects (SMILY stick figure drawings!) 2. Compare, identify, and analyze attributes to develop the vocabulary needed to describe geometric shapes (the head is down; the arms are up; the leg is bent) 3. Put shapes together to form other shapes
Describe spatial relationships	1. Use spatial vocabulary (left, right, above, below) 2. Participate in group activities based on the concepts of space and location (yoga!) 3. Describe location and movement using common language and geometric vocabulary (how to do poses)
Apply transformations and use symmetry to analyzemathematical situations.	1. Investigate the symmetry of two-dimensional shapes (by folding or cutting paper: making books) 2. Create simple symmetrical shapes and pictures 3. Use materials to create shapes that have symmetry
Use visualization, spatial reasoning and geometric modeling to solve problems	1. Describe how to get from one location to another (how to move from one posture to another) 2. Participate in activities to develop mental visualization and spatial memory (SMILY Dot Books) 3. Select and use visualization skills to create mental images of geometric shapes (matching, sequencing)

Table 19: Physical Education Benchmarks

STANDARD	BENCHMARK = SMILY APPROACH
Apply movement concepts and principles to the learning and development of motor skills.	1. Demonstrate concepts of body, effort, space and relationships in movement. 2. Demonstrate motor learning concepts in increasingly complex situations 3. Demonstrate elements of fundamental and specialized movement skills
Exhibit knowledge and ability to participate in an active lifestyle	1. Participate regularly in health related physical activities for enjoyment 2. Identify the benefits gained from regular physical activity
Achieve and maintain a health-enhancing level of physical fitness.	1. Match different types of physical activities with the related physical fitness components (balance, strength, coordination) 2. Participate in physical activities in a variety of settings
Demonstrate responsibile personal and social behavior in physical activity settings.	1. Work cooperatively and productively with a partner or small group 2. Work independently and on-task for short periods of time 3. Recognize classroom and activity rules
Understand and erspect difference among people in physical activity settings.	1. Explore self-awareness through participation in physical activity (YOGA!) 2. Recognize the talents that different people
Understand and respect differences amoung people in physical activity settings.	1. Identify physical activities that are enjoyable 2. Practice physical activities to increase skills 3. Interact with others while participating in activity 4. Use physical activity as means for self-expression social interaction

Table 20: Arts Performance Benchmarks

STANDARD	BENCHMARK = SMILY APPROACH
Learn and develop the essential skills and technical demands of dance, music, drama and visual arts.	1. Accurately demonstrate basic locomotor movements 2. Demonstrate kinesthetic (sensory) awareness, focus and concentration, and accuracy while moving to various rhythms. 3. Show the concepts of personal space and general space, working alone, with a partner, and in a group 4. Sing and speak using appropriate vocal techniques while maintaining a steady beat 5. Explore through movement simple rhythm patterns 6. Use body and voice to portray characters that contribute to the action of a story 7. Improvise dialogue to tell stories 8. Participate in the process of making art by using different materials
Use dance, music, drama and visual arts to express ideas.	1. Recognize music as a type of language capable of expressing ideas. 2. Describe the moods or emotional qualities of different kinds of performances (characters in stories)
Demonstrate an understanding of the dynamics of the creative process.	1. Improvise completion of a given rhythmic or melodic phrase 2. Understand that there are multiple ways in which a phrase may be completed
Integrate understanding of visual and performing arts by seeking connections and parallels among arts disciplines as well as other content areas.	1. Collaborate to plan, rehearse and perform (routine) 2. Compare the ways in which repetition, balance, symmetry and pattern occur in content areas other than art (compare physical poses with their characters, drawings and names) 3. Use a piece of art to produce a writing piece (use stick figures to make a SMILY book)

SECTION SIX

Special Education:

Therapists & Teachers

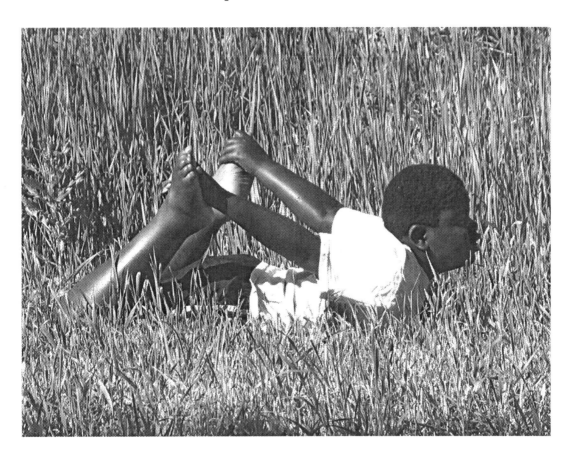

The Individualized Education Plan

Children receiving Special Education services have annually updated Individualized Education Plans (IEP's), which contain their present levels of performance as well as goals for the next 12 months. Across states and school systems, Special Education Departments must handle their IEP's according to their local requirements and standards. Trends fluctuate, and professionals learn to use changing terms to refer to commonly used methods, principles and childhood conditions. For example, there are varying definitions for goals, objectives, performance standards, or benchmarks. Teachers and therapists from different districts are sometimes directed to write these "goals" in divergent ways, as school systems work to stay current and in compliance with state regulations. Regardless of the specific requirements in your district, SMILY is appropriate and applicable. In short, use the language your directors are asking you to use. Call them objectives or benchmarks or standards, whatever fits. Then use them in the IEP to set the course for providing services to your students and meeting their individual needs.

Now a special note for Special Education teachers, also known as Resource teachers in some districts. The textual information in this book is intended to provide you with ample justification for using the SMILY program as a Special Education service. Always keep in mind the benefits, the components of learning needed for success in school, and the research sections. Look over the preceding section of "Educational Benchmarks" for evidence that the SMILY approach does address fundamental academic concepts. You can use these examples as goals or objectives in your students IEP's and be confident that you are meeting the needs of your students through the SMILY program. Or, review your own state standards with SMILY in mind and choose similar benchmarks that address the same concepts.

Remember that you can offer SMILY sessions in your classroom as educationally relevant lessons. You can also work in conjunction with therapists, following the multi-disciplinary or team approach to delivering Special Education service. You can even work together with Regular Education teachers, offering SMILY sessions as inclusion based activities. (Refer to the Introduction section).

Therapy Goals: OT, PT and SLP

As an Occupational Therapist, I understand the importance of linking our treatment sessions with specified goals to be sure we are meeting the individual needs of students. Ancillary services of Occupational, Speech and Physical Therapy are intended to support a student's progress through the educational system and to enhance the individualized services he receives through Special Education. I am aware of some school districts where therapists are no longer writing their own separate goals. Instead, they are asked to direct their services toward the components needed for success in key academic areas. In this case, therapists are working to meet educational benchmarks like the ones in the preceding section.

Therapy serves to enhance the necessary components of learning. Use of the SMILY program is a perfect way to support academic progress in this way. Other therapists are working in a strong team environment, working together to meet common or shared goals across disciplines. With this approach, SMILY is a wonderful way to provide co-treatment sessions and support progress in overlapping areas.

With regard to the IEP, many therapists are concerned that yoga may not be a sufficient means of addressing a child's goals. It may not be immediately clear exactly how yoga can meet stated therapy goals. This is one reason why I designed SMILY to be so much more than just yoga for kids: so that it fully supports the development of fundamental skills related to learning. Perhaps a therapist is aware of the many benefits of yoga and comfortable using it, but is unsure exactly how to write goals to support that modality. My response is: look carefully at the benefits of yoga; the principles of Sensory Integration; the components of learning; and the research sections of this book. There is plenty of support in this text to help you justify the use of yoga with children within the IEP itself as well as with administrators.

The next step is: take another look at the current goals you have already written for the children on your caseload. Consider each goal and ask yourself if any portion of the SMILY program helps build skills related to that goal. Chances are quite good that you can simply keep the exact goals you have established for your students, and SMILY will allow you to continue working on them. In this case, just consider SMILY to be another therapeutic modality like any other (only lots better!). Don't get hung up on wondering if yoga meets their needs, or addresses therapy goals. We can easily show that it does. So you can use it with confidence.

Still, isn't it just nice sometimes to see some examples? Yes! So, I am including a few sample goals that I have used in different IEP's over the years. I never cease to be amazed how many areas of development the SMILY program supports. When I am writing goals for my students, I am not necessarily thinking about making the goals fit the SMILY program. First of all, I am writing goals with the student's educational progress in mind. As it turns out, just about any goal I write can be addressed through SMILY because it is so widely encompassing. Goal writing just really isn't that big of an issue with regard to using SMILY, because it all works! Table 21 provides some examples to help you get started - over time you will feel increasingly comfortable with the process.

Table 21: Sample Therapy Goals for OT, PT & SLP

POSTURAL CONTROL - PT and OT Goals

- Stand on one leg for 5 (or 10) seconds without twisting trunk, waving arms or stepping down.

- Maintain both flexion and extension postures for 5 (or 10) seconds without stopping.

- Smoothly and accurately transition from one physical posture to the next without losing balance.

- Maintain upright seated posture on floor without support of hands for 30 seconds.

PERCEPTUAL SKILLS – PT and OT Goals

- Use drawings to correctly imitate postures with accurate spatial orientation of body parts.

- Sequence a series of physical postures in correct order using visual memory, motor planning and motor memory skills.

- Organize a series of drawings into correct sequential order.

- Correctly match printed words with drawings of physical postures.

SENSORY ORGANIZATION: ATTENTION AND BEHAVIOR – PT and OT Goals

- Maintain steady visual gaze upon relevant object for minimum of 2 minutes without distraction.

- Effectively practice deep belly breathing for at least 10 breaths, independently and without stopping.

- Maintain supine relaxation posture for at least 3 minutes without moving or talking.

- Participate in functional activities at table top for at least 10 minutes without leaving the table.

- Demonstrate independent work behavior by organizing materials and staying on task for at least 10 minutes with no more than one verbal cue

- Participate in structured group activity for at least 10 (or 20) minutes without leaving the group.

FINE MOTOR / GROSS MOTOR – PT and OT Goals

- Maintain weight bearing posture on open hands for at least 10 seconds without collapsing.

- Exhibit efficient use of crayons, pencils and markers for 10 minutes.

- Accurately trace shapes with no more than 2 (or 3) errors per activity.

- Maintain upright seated posture at table for at least 5 minutes without slumping or propping body on elbows.

- Complete fine motor project within allotted time frame with minimal cueing

- Accurately cut around small pictures using correct scissor grip, with no more than 2 (or 3) errors per activity.

AUDITORY PROCESSING - OT and SLP Goals

- Follow 2 step (or 3 step) commands correctly and independently.

- Accurately repeat complete sentences verbally.

- Respond appropriately and accurately to questions about stories/songs.

- Respond correctly to verbal directions to change physical positions.

- Correctly retell a story by stating 2 or 3 main ideas independently.

- Verbally sequence song lyrics correctly (one or two verses).

FUNCTIONAL LANGUAGE - OT and SLP Goals

- Consistently use appropriate greetings when arriving and departing.

- Exhibit awareness of suitable turn taking skills in conversation.

- Ask relevant questions that relate to the song or task at hand.

- Offer verbal answers to questions from adults with reasonable accuracy.

- Demonstrate ability to stay on current topic for at least 10 minutes.

THERAPY LOG TABLE (Table 22 - reproducible)

Routine_____   Start Date(s)_____

Time/Group_____   Finish Date(s)_____

Date   Student(s)   Goals/Progress/Notes

SECTION SEVEN:

How to Teach Children

Breathing, Relaxation & Postures

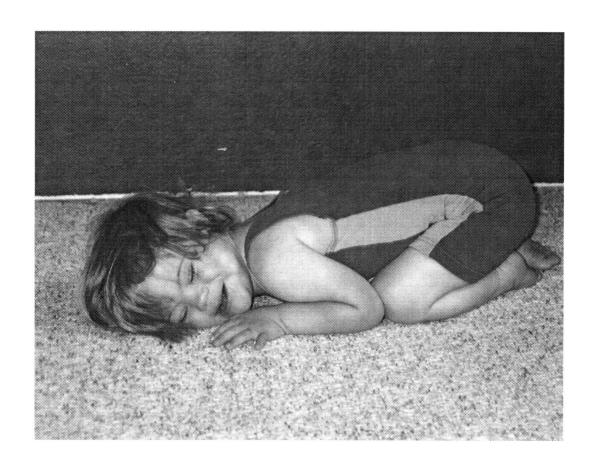

Breathing

Any true yoga practice must include an awareness or perception of the breath. See Table 23 for the benefits of deepened breathing; see how they relate to classroom performance.

Table 23: Benefits of Breathing

Balances nervous system: allows for relaxation and calm focus
Increases oxygen to the brain: Improved cognitive function
Balance the hemispheres of the brain: Promotes complex functions
Creates flexibility and efficiency of muscles: Greater endurance/less fatigue
Equalizes levels of alertness: Energizes lethargic child or calms overly active
Improves overall health: slower heart rate; less tension; better sleep and digestion; improves immune system
Gives a sense of personal control, peace and confidence

TEACHING TIPS:

1) Have kids lying on their backs with knees bent. This relaxes the back and neck, and allows the diaphragm to move more freely in the torso.

2) Say, "Breathe in like you're smelling your most favorite food" and "Breathe out like you're blowing out all the candles on your birthday cake"

3) Say, "When you breathe in, your tummy goes up" and "When you breathe out, your tummy goes back down"

4) After asking permission, place your hand on the child's belly. Say, "Breathe in and make my hand go up" and "Breathe out and make my hand go down"

5) Have the children watch you breathing while lying on your back. Tell them to watch how your belly goes up and down.

6) If it's comfortable, the children can also try placing their hands on your belly, or even on each other's, to feel the up and down movement while breathing.

Relaxation

Being able to practice some form of relaxation is a highly valuable tool for everyone in this busy world, including children. As adults we might sometimes forget that children also experience stress in their lives and very much need to be taught how to release tension. The ability to truly relax is a remarkable advantage that can greatly affect how well a child can learn in the educational environment. Table 24 lists some of the benefits we can all experience:

Table 24: Benefits of Relaxation

Allows brain time to process information so that deeper learning can occur.
Integration of physical activity so that motor planning can become motor memory skills.
Overall stress reduction – lowering of stress related biochemicals in the nervous system.
Enhanced attention/concentration and memory.
Improved immune system function; fewer days absent from school due to illness
Improved sleep – less fatigue, better alertness
Improved digestion and assimilation of nutrients for better physical, emotional and mental functions
Greater self-esteem, well-being and confidence.

TEACHING TIPS:

1) Be consistent: ALWAYS include the relaxation portion in every session!
2) Call it "Dreamer" and say, "Pretend you are going to sleep".
3) Instruct , "No moving, no talking, no noises" (repeat if necessary).
4) Model relaxation by lying down with the children. Turn off lights.
5) Use a timer with a beeper. Let kids say how many minutes they want.

6) Use blankets to cover/wrap snugly; or 3 to 4 pound rice bags on legs or belly.

Yoga Poses

For anyone, the practice of yoga involves imitation of posture. Some children are naturally more adept at this than others. It is important to bear in mind our discussion of Gardner's Multiple Intelligences when teaching yoga poses to children. As you get to know your students more, you will come to know what their relative learning strengths are. Some children will imitate the postures better by watching you demonstrate, rather than looking at the stick figure drawings, which require more abstract spatial relationships.

For those that have a difficult time with motor planning, you may need to break down the steps of how to move the body into a pose, or transition from one posture to the next. In this case, use clear language to describe the movements. For example, to verbalize the Wind Pose in the Garden routine say: "Pat your right leg…Step all the way back with your right foot…Now bend your left knee and turn your body to face the other wall…Pick up your arms…Good! Now you're the Wind!"

It is important that you as the teacher fully know how to do the poses and have practiced them yourself before beginning each new routine. As you do the postures, think about the movements required to get into each pose and the vocabulary needed to describe that process. Be prepared to verbally instruct any pose in case you want to make any corrections to your students' imitation of posture.

Of course, for children who have delays in auditory processing and have a difficult time following spoken directions, this approach will not work. Under this circumstance, encourage them to focus their visual attention on how you are physically demonstrating the pose. Even better, instruct them to watch how one of the other children is doing the posture, which serves as an excellent model. If auditory processing and motor planning are both challenging for the child, first allow him to approximate the posture as best he can. Praise him for that effort, then ask if you can help. Give clear, unambiguous hands-on assistance by placing your hands at the most obvious body part that looks to be the furthest from performing the pose correctly. This may mean getting the student to separate his feet more, or bend his knee, or change the position of his arms. Do not try to fix every little thing about the pose. Pick just one or maybe two corrections, and stick with those until he does them independently. This may take a few repetitions but it will improve! Remember to focus on staying safe and aiming for accuracy, but also allow the child to feel good about the effort he is making.

And now a word about apparent lack of effort. It is important to remember that a sensory-motor experience such as yoga can be extremely challenging for some children. There will be times when they need a break and maybe don't want to try so hard. Sometimes it is necessary to allow this because the sensory-motor system is feeling overwhelmed. In such cases, break the activity down into smaller packages. If the student is singing but not doing the poses, focus more on the song and pair it with simple rhythmic clapping or crossing midline movements.

It is not necessary, or even possible sometimes, to pair the music with the movement, and so we have to pick one. If he is doing the movements but not really singing, simplify the language by just calling out the names of the poses instead of singing the whole song. Stay tuned in with the challenge level, keep it as "just right" as you can without causing undo stress. Because the session is taking place in a group format, just try to think of creative solutions to modify the music and movement components so that all the children have various options to "up-grade" or "down-grade" their experience as needed.

Of course, sometimes lack of participation can be due to an internal emotional state, lack of interest, or a specific behavioral issue. In these cases, I have found the best approach is to first of all set very clear boundaries as much as possible. Use clear, simple language such as, "This is what we're doing today" or "You are here to do yoga with us". Tell them in no uncertain terms exactly what is expected of them and hold firm to that every single time. The use of clearly marked physical boundaries is also extremely helpful. I am fortunate to have actual yoga mats in my therapy room, and one of my rules is that each child is required to stay on his mat until we have finished the routine and Dreamer. You can also use tape on the floor, or other types of mats such as carpet squares or colored shapes to mark a child's spot.

Again, consistent praise is vital to participation. Here are some "Words of Encouragement" I often use to keep the performance level up:

- Show me how strong you are!
- That's perfect! You look awesome!
- Good job, keep going!
- Come on, only you can control your body!
- That's great! I knew you could do it!
- You are really good at this!
- Look at you! Excellent! Right on! Terrific! Etc.
- This is your job, it's up to you, make it really good!
- You can do this, show me what you can do!
- Now do your very best!
- Show me how tall you are!
- That's the best yet!

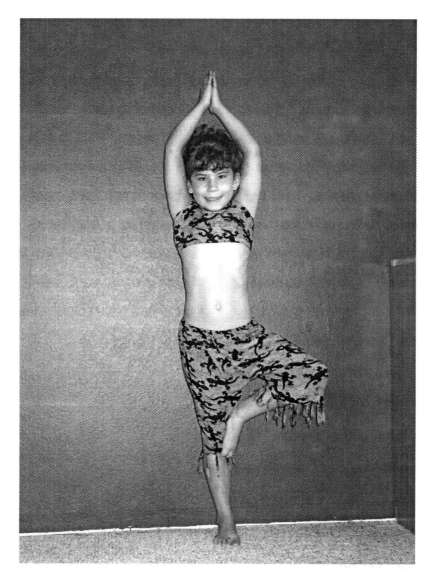

Balancing Postures

One legged balancing poses often present a special challenge for many children. Improvement can take awhile, but balance does come along with repetition and practice. Definitely keep working at it, it will pay off! Here are some ways to help children develop their balance skills.

TEACHING TIPS:

1) **NUMBER ONE!!** The visual system makes up about one-third of our sense of balance. It is very important to teach children to focus their visual gaze on an unmoving spot in order to steady their balance.

A) I make sure every child I work with sees me do the following demonstration at least once because it really, really helps:

First the group attempts to do a balancing pose. Try it on both sides. If anyone struggles, stop and get their attention. If they are quite young, ask if anyone knows what "balancing" is, and describe it as "not falling over". You can give an example such as riding on a bicycle or skateboard. Tell them, "Here we are balancing on one leg, and not falling over".

Ask everyone to stand where they can see your eyes. Do the same balancing pose and move your eyes all around the room, twist your body and wave your arms and step down out of the pose (as if you're falling over). Say, "What happens when I move my eyes all around?". They will tell you that you fall over. Do it a second time. Then say, "Watch me now, I'm going to keep my eyes on one spot and not move my eyes". Do the pose again, keeping your eyes very steady on one point. Ask them, "Now what happens?". They will see that you are keeping your balance.

At the next subsequent session, when the group comes to the balancing posture in the routine, ask them, "What do we do with our eyes?". They will say, "Keep them in one place!"

B) Especially with younger children, it is very helpful to provide them with the specific place to focus their visual gaze. I like to use the chalkboard (or dry erase) and write the letter of their first name with a circle around it. As much as possible, put it right in front of them so they can be looking straight ahead, and at eye level. Usually the student will want to write the letter themselves, and this might be an exception where they are allowed to come off their mat to write on the board. If you are using a wall, tape a piece of paper up with their letter on it.

2) Hands-on Assistance. If holding they eyes steady is not enough, or your student has great difficulty focusing his visual attention, you may need to provide physical assistance. It is important to ask permission first. Ask if you can help, or at the very least tell the child that you are going to help him do the pose with your hands. Sometimes this may feel like you are practically holding the child up, but that's okay. Say, "Hey, I'm doing all the work here. Help me! Try to hold your body up...That's better...that's it!" There are two primary ways of giving hands-on help during balancing postures:

a) For children really having the most difficulty and needing the greatest amount of input: Stand behind the child and place both your hands right on top of his hips, at the top of the pelvis (iliac crest). Use a fairly firm rather than a light touch, and press straight down towards the floor so that he can connect from the hips down to his heels (= joint approximation). Instruct him to hold his arms up on his own in the pose.

b) For children who are progressing in their balance skills but still need a little help staying upright: Stand in front of the child and hold either one or both hands. This may mean the arms are not doing the pose; that's okay for now.

3) Other tips to share with your students:
- "Squeeze the muscles of your legs...squeeze, squeeze!"
- "Keep your knee straight" or "Push your knee back"
- "Pretend your feet are growing roots right down into the ground"
- "Let's see if we can all stay up while we count to ten"
- Older students can count by ordinals (two's, five's, ten's, etc.)

When teaching yoga to children, remember that some will need lots of repetition, verbal cues, physical assistance and encouragement. Stay with the practice and I guarantee that over time you will begin to see the benefits. Watch for progress and be sure to document improvements as they occur!

SECTION EIGHT:

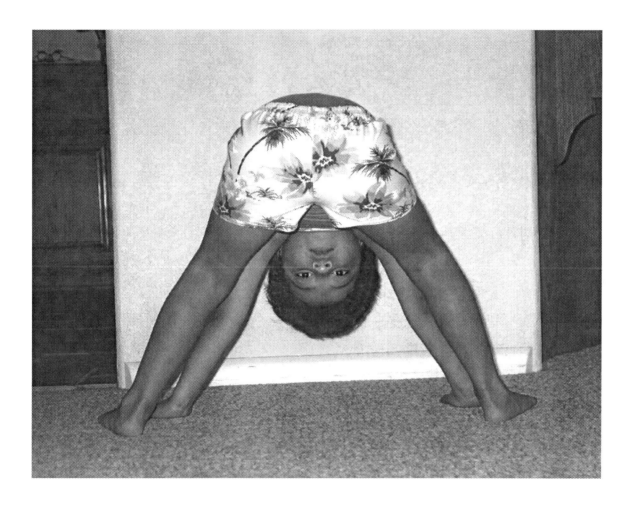

S.M.I.L.Y. Routines & Materials

Two S.M.I.L.Y. Companion CD's are available providing a soundtrack of songs and narrated posture instruction for each routine. Please see the last page of the book for ordering information.

April Merrilee

The 8 S.M.I.L.Y. Routines

1   The Magic Garden

2   Tom Cat

3   Guess Who

4   Old Man Winter

5   Going On Safari

6   The Butterflies

7   Swimming Lessons

8   Mama Duck

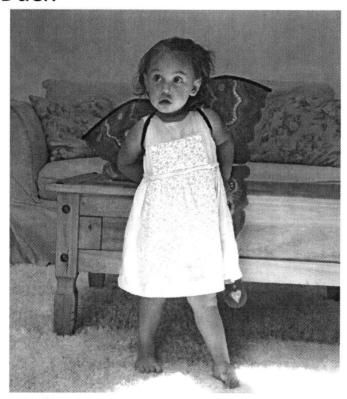

Lesson Materials

Materials are presented in the following order for each S.M.I.L.Y. routine.

1. INTRODUCTORY STORY WITH LANGUAGE HIGHLIGHTS
2. SONG LYRICS
3. PHOTOGRAPHS OF CHILDREN, ALL 8 POSES
4. LARGE STICK FIGURE DRAWINGS – IN SEQUENCE, 1 PER PAGE, 8 PAGES
5. DOT-TO-DOT DRAWINGS – 2 PER PAGE, 4 PAGES PER ROUTINE
6. STICK FIGURE DRAWINGS FOR "ANIMAL PICTURES" – 2 PAGES
7. STICK FIGURE DRAWINGS FOR MATCHING – ALL 8 ON ONE PAGE
8. NAMES OF POSES FOR MATCHING GAMES – ALL 8 ON ONE PAGE
9. SMALL STICK FIGURES FOR SENTENCE WORKSHEETS – ALL 8
10. SENTENCE WORKSHEETS: BASIC AND CHALLENGE ON ONE PAGE
11. SPELLING BOOKS – 4 PER PAGE, 2 PAGES PER ROUTINE

SMILY Activities

After the music and movement portion of a SMILY session, the following fine motor, visual motor and visual perceptual tasks can be set up as the final adaptive response or outcome. Feel free to spread these activities out over more than one session if the children in your group are slower to complete. It can actually be a good learning practice to keep their unfinished material to be finished at the next session. This teaches students how to maintain effort for an on-going project, enhancing the qualities of consistency, persistence and patience!

I have presented them in the order I usually prefer, but it is fine to do them in a different sequence. Usually, when I introduce a brand new routine for the very first time, we focus on learning the story, song and poses and do not include an activity for the first session. It takes a little longer to get through the music and movement portions the first couple of times. After that, the children are generally starting to get the hang of it and then we have more time to devote to the educational activities.

When teachers and/or parents also participate in the full session, there is the option of sending unfinished work to be completed later in the classroom or as homework. All the materials needed for each lesson are included in the section titled, "The SMILY Routines". You may copy them for therapy/teaching purposes.

NOTE: Remember that each and every session includes:

- First few minutes on back for belly breathing
- Full routine of 3 repetitions. Third time without singing, do poses quietly
- DREAMER. Please be sure to always include relaxation
- Choose one of the following activities, using the reproducible materials found in the following section (Section Eight).

<u>Session 1</u>   Tell introductory story; sit in an upright, cross-legged position. ("criss cross applesauce") Tell the title of the story/song. Be dramatic! Teach song lyrics and melody. Keep stick figure drawings out of sight at first. Define new vocabulary. Pair song with rhythmic clapping or simple movements to cross the midline.

Introduce large stick figure drawings, hanging the series of 8 poses from left to right on wall. I like to staple each page onto a piece of construction paper for visual contrast and greater durability. Always have these figures displayed in this same manner for every SMILY session. Practice yoga poses separately from singing, one or two repetitions to start. Teach safety and accuracy as applicable.

Option: Google search for images of the animals represented by the stick figure drawings, and print the pictures prior to the first session. Especially helpful for introducing more unusual animals such as flamingo, peacock and ostrich. Also nice to use with younger or lower functioning children for matching games.

Option: Print song lyrics onto posterboard for display during sessions. Or use copy machine to enlarge lyrics from text of this book.

<u>Sessions 2 and 3</u>   Review story, ask what the students remember. Ask basic comprehension questions about what happens in the story.

Children make their own **SMILY Dot Books** using dot to dot worksheets. (Make enough copies for everyone). Children trace both the pose and its name on each page. Be sure to include the "kids lyrics page" in the back of each book. Make a book cover using construction paper following the sample provided, including the title of the story and the child's name. Work on sequencing skills by having each child put drawings into right order. Encourage children to use their books to practice at home, and to show teachers and parents. (Save pages for students between sessions until project completed.)

Option: Pay attention to how your students complete each dot to dot figure. It can be very informative to watch how they connect the body parts, as a clue to their own sense of body scheme or awareness. You may choose to direct the activity by instructing them to: "Draw the head first and the body next. Then put on the legs, and put the arms on last"

<u>Session 4</u> **SMILY Animal Pictures:** use the two pages that have the stick figure drawings, 4 to a page, without smily faces. Instruct students to draw on these figures and make them look like the animals they are. Assist them by talking about what body parts the various animals would need. For example, the cat needs whiskers and ears and a tail...the cow needs spots and an udder, etc. etc. Encourage kids to get creative. One preschooler put a crown on her frog! Other kids like to add other objects to their drawings, such as carrots for the horse, or mud for the pig. You can have a lot of fun with this one!

<u>Sessions 5 and 6</u> Children make **SMILY Game Pieces** using worksheets that have all 8 poses on one page, and the sheets that have the 8 names on one page. Each child makes his own set. Glue these two worksheets onto pieces of construction paper in two different colors (one color for poses, another color for names). Cut each sheet into 8 game pieces for a total of 16. Fold and staple construction paper

into two separate envelopes for the game pieces (one for poses, one for names). As much as possible, let your students do the folding. Put their names on the envelopes and save for the next session.

Option: Before gluing and cutting, use bright colored markers to trace over stick figure drawings. Can also practice copy skills by having students write the names just below the printed version on the page. This will help develop visual motor and visual discrimination skills.

<u>Session 7</u> (1) **Matching Game** using SMILY Game Pieces from envelopes. Each student plays with his own set of game pieces. For inclusion, divide into smaller groups of 4 or 5 students each. Everyone turns all pieces face down, with poses to one side and names to the other. Go around taking turns within each group. Turn over a pose, then a name. If they match, keep the pair face up as a "win". If not place them both face down again. Cue your students to remember where they placed them for the next turn. (2) **Sequencing Game**. Put game pieces into correct sequential order (both names and poses).

Option: Practice sequencing without looking at display of large stick figure drawings (cover or remove prior to activity)

<u>Session 8</u> **SMILY Sentence Sheets**, using worksheet of very small stick figure drawings with blank lines, and the appropriate sentence sheet for each routine. There are two levels of sentence sheets: (1) **Basic copying** for younger or lower level children OR (2) **Challenge sentences** that give clues about the animal or object so students have to match them. Provide students with the sentence sheet that best meets or challenges their skill levels. Note the figures and sentences are not in correct sequential order for the challenge sentences!

Sessions 9 and 10 Make **SMILY Spelling Books**, using worksheets that read, "Dd is for _____". Note these pages are not in the same sequential order but are mixed up to increase attention to detail. Cue students to trace the dot to dot version of the upper case and lower case letters. Use worksheet of 8 names as a guide to fill in boxes with correct spelling. Also helps with copy skills as well as regulating sizing and spacing. Cut into pages, and help students arrange pages back into correct sequential order. Staple into book form with another construction paper book cover. Include title and student's name on cover.

Option: After stapling the book, provide students with worksheet that has the 8 stick figure poses on one page. On the back of each spelling page, the student can either: (1) Draw the appropriate stick figure to develop visual motor skills OR (2) Cut and glue from the worksheet. Hint: glue sticks are best, less wet!

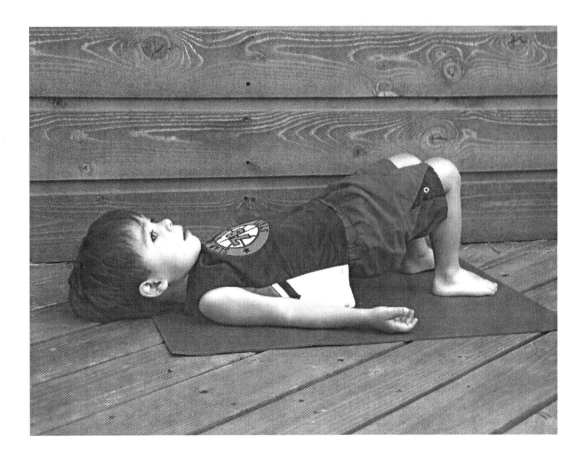

PRESCHOOLERS - ACTIVITY SUGGESTIONS

Because some of the SMILY functional activities are not truly age appropriate for all preschoolers, I change my approach somewhat at the preschool setting. I tend to do the SMILY program for just a few weeks with preschoolers, and then move on to a new one, rather than working on it for several weeks as I might do with older students. Here are some suggestions for fine motor/visual motor activities:

1. Sensory Art Projects: From a kids' coloring book, find a picture of an animal in the story/song - preferably the main character but any animal will work. For example, for Guess Who you can use a pig, and create a wig for him, which follows the story line. Provide a variety of tactile art supplies and use glue to decorate with: sequins, beads, yarn, feathers, cotton balls, etc.

2. SMILY Dot Books (see sessions 2 and 3 above) depending upon the ages and abilities of your students. This activity may need to be introduced a few times before some children understand the concept of connecting dots. Instruct them to trace and show them how. Even if they don't quite get it right, I feel this is still a very good visual motor activity for young children to experience. Do make sure the large stick figure drawings are visibly on display.

3. SMILY Animal Pictures: (see session 4 above.)

4 and 5. Matching Games: have children create game pieces as one session (see sessions 5 and 6 above). Teach them that one set (on one color of construction paper) is the poses and the other set (on another color) is the names. Then the next week, modify so that instead of taking turns, each child uses his own game piece individually but simultaneously with everyone in the group, to find its matching counterpart. Instruct them to first look at the color set of poses, and then to find a specific animal pose. I recommend going in the same order as the song/routine.

Then have everyone in the group find the matching word from that color set. "Now put your matching pair into your envelope." And repeat! Again, make sure the large stick figure drawings are visibly on display.

6. Other related projects: Modifying pictures from coloring books, make **masks:** color and cut out, then glue on to construction paper and secure with yarn; or **puppets:** use small brown paper bags and pictures of animals heads/faces; glue upper face onto bottom section of bag and the animal's mouth below that on side of bag, so that when child puts hand into upside down bag, the mouth moves.

ROUTINE # 1: THE MAGIC GARDEN

Once upon a time there was a big lonely field near a small town in the country. No plants grew there except some sad looking brown grass. No animals ever came to sit or sleep or eat in the field. Not even the wind or the rain ever came to visit! It was a very lonely field. One day, in the summer time, what a surprise! A man drove up on a brand new yellow tractor. He said he wanted to grow a garden in the field, and it was the perfect time to plant the seeds. This man had never been a farmer before. The people in the little town just laughed at his idea of growing a garden in that big lonely field where nothing ever happened. They laughed and said, "He'll NEVER get anything to grow out there, nothing will ever happen out in that sad lonely field!" The man heard them laughing but it did not bother him because, guess what? He knew something they didn't know. He had something special to help grow a garden, and nobody knew about it. What do you think he had?

Well, I'll tell you what it was: he had a very special MAGIC WAND And he planned to use it to make the garden grow. But he couldn't let the town people see him using the wand. So, during the day he worked at plowing the earth into neat rows and planting the seeds. Let me see you do those things! (Imitate actions of plowing and planting with hands.) At night, when nobody was watching, the man would bring out his magic wand and wave it all over the field! Let me see you wave your magic wand! See, this man knew that a lonely garden would never grow. So he asked the magic wand to bring some animals to visit, and for some wind and rain to help things grow, too. He did this every night for a whole week, and when he was done he said, "There! Now I know some magic will happen in this field. I will pick my vegetables this fall, and come winter the field can rest for a while. Then, I can tell everybody in town about everything that happened while my magic garden was growing."

LANGUAGE HIGHLIGHTS - GARDEN SONG

- Prepositions (over, through, above, on, in, from, around, with)
- Irregular verbs – past tense (fell, blew, flew, sat, slept, ate, drove, grew, taught)
- Conjugate verbs (grow, growing, grew)
- Initial /p/ sound
- /r/ sound – initial and blends
- Final /ing/ sound

THE MAGIC GARDEN

Sung to the tune of " Row, Row, Row Your Boat"

First verse:

Rain falls over the field
Will the garden grow?
Magic is happening,
We just have to believe
This is what we know

Wind blows through the field
Will the garden grow?
Magic is happening,
We just have to believe
This is what we know

Crow flies above the field
(repeat above lines)

Turkey sits with the field…

Possum sleeps on the field…

Pig eats from the field…

Farmer drives around the field

Pumpkin shines in the field …

Second Verse:

Rain fell over the field
Yes, the garden grew
Magic was happening
Because we did believe
This is always true.

Wind blew through the field
Yes, the garden grew
Magic was happening
Because we did believe
This is always true.

Crow flew above the field
(repeat above lines)

Turkey sat with the field…

Possum slept on the field…

Pig ate from the field…

Farmer drove around the field…

Pumpkin shone in the field

Between verses: Explain that the garden does not grow all year. In the winter, nothing grows. We can tell the story about what happended in the garden while it was growing (past tense verbs). Let's sing about it!

April Merrilee

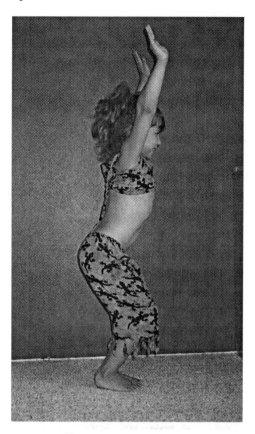
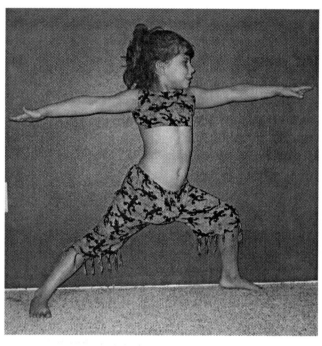
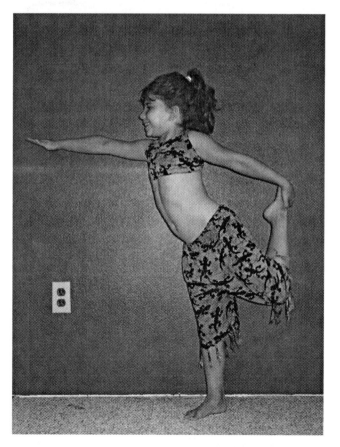
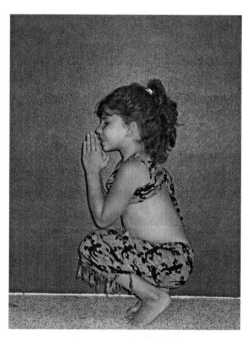

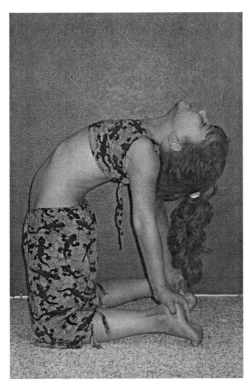
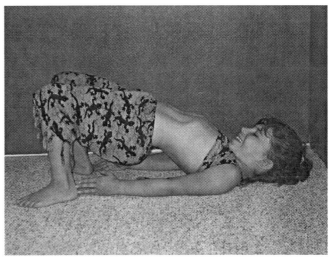
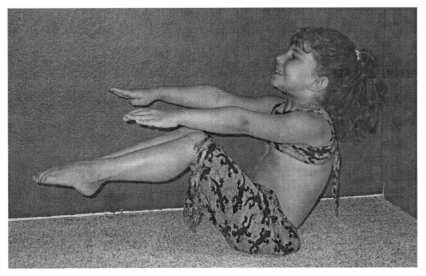
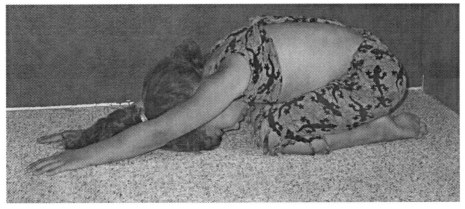

April Merrilee

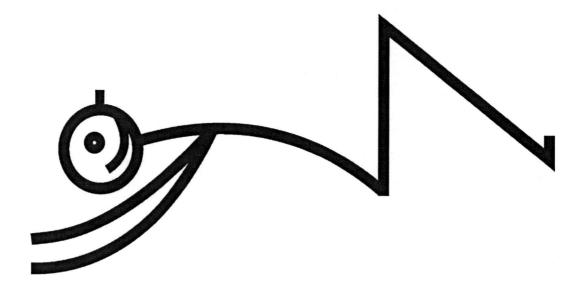

rain

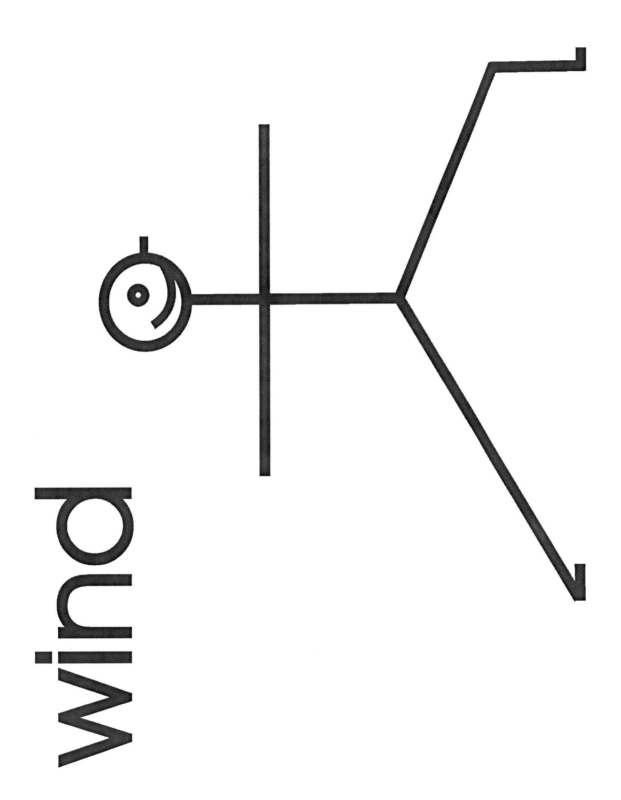

April Merrilee

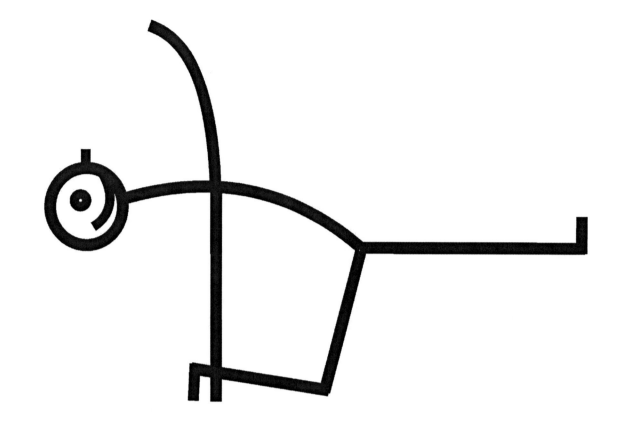

crow

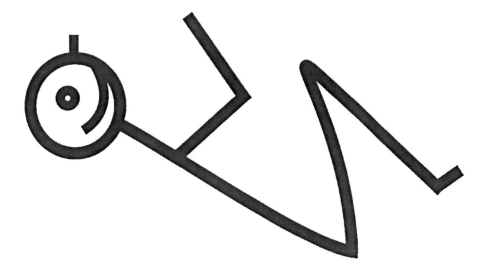

turkey

April Merrilee

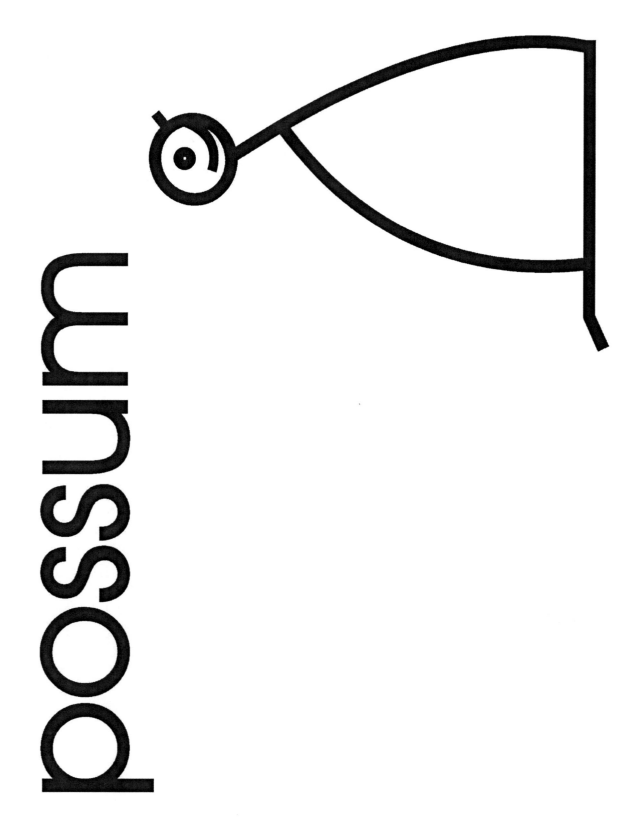

S.M.I.L.Y

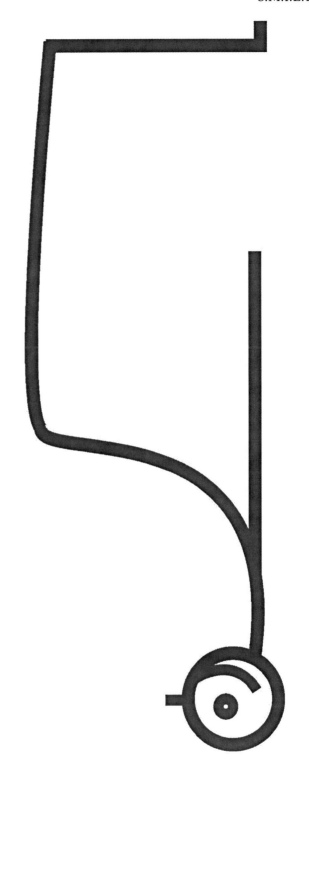

pig

April Merrilee

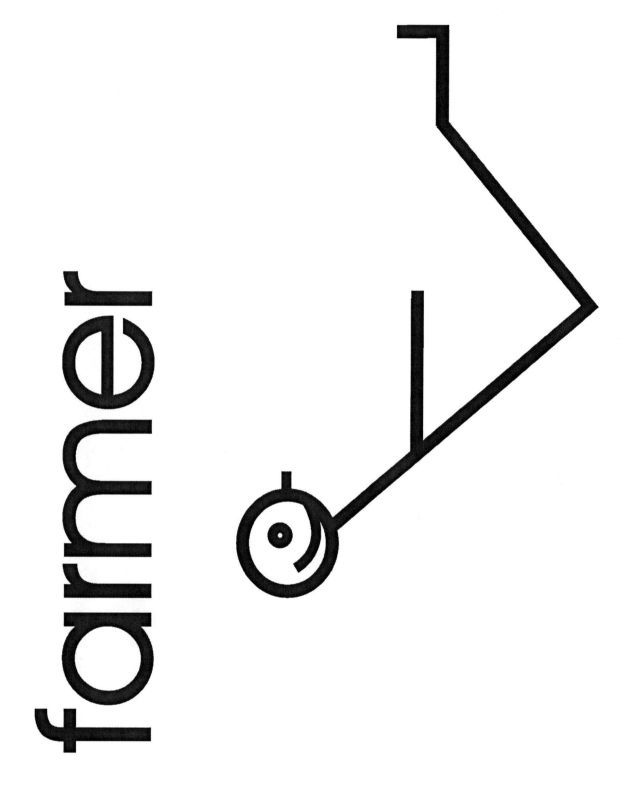

pumpkin

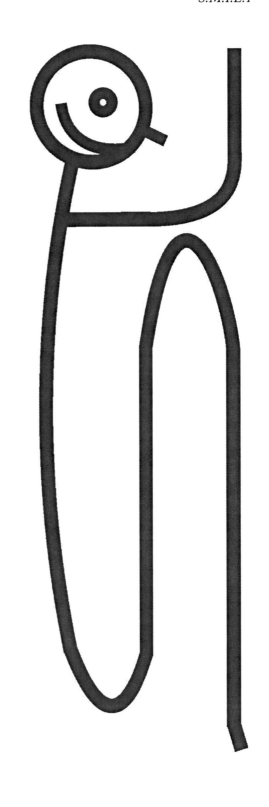

April Merrilee

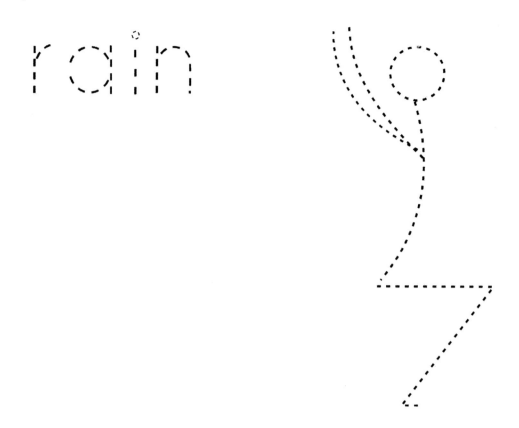

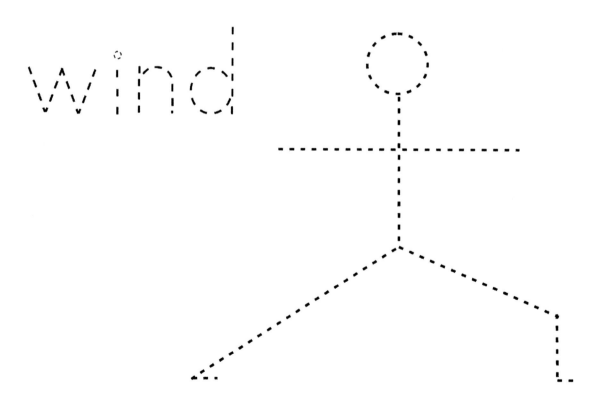

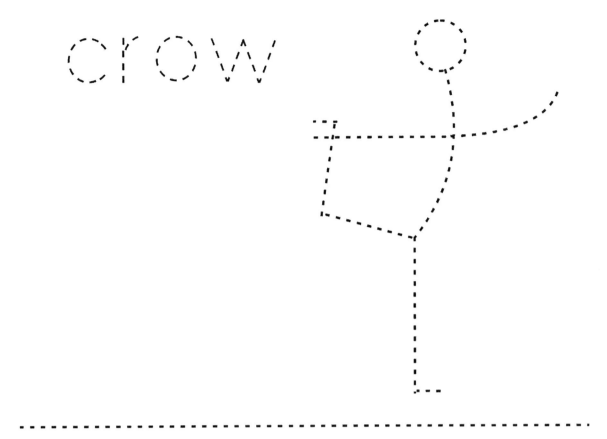

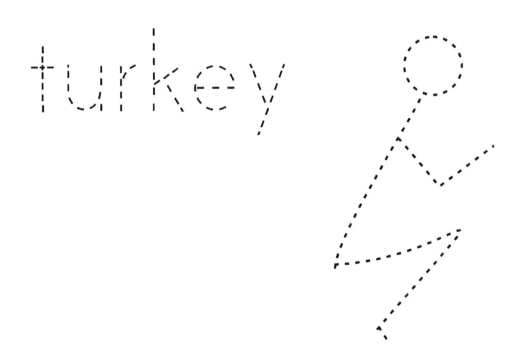

April Merrilee

possum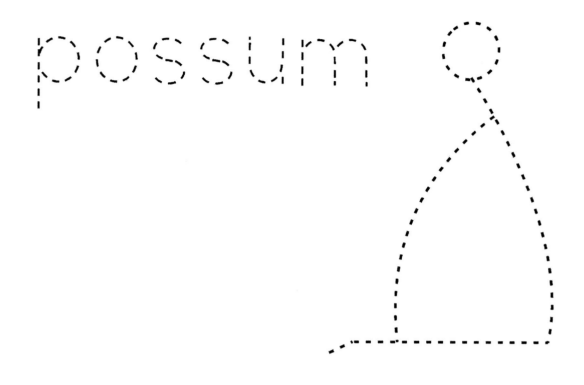

---

pig

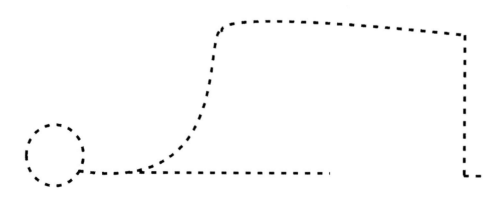

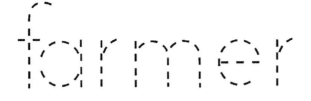

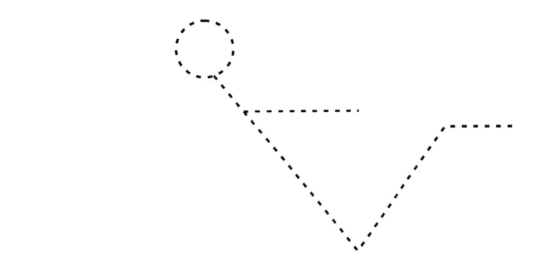

pumpkin

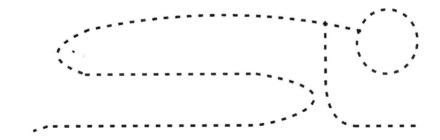

April Merrilee

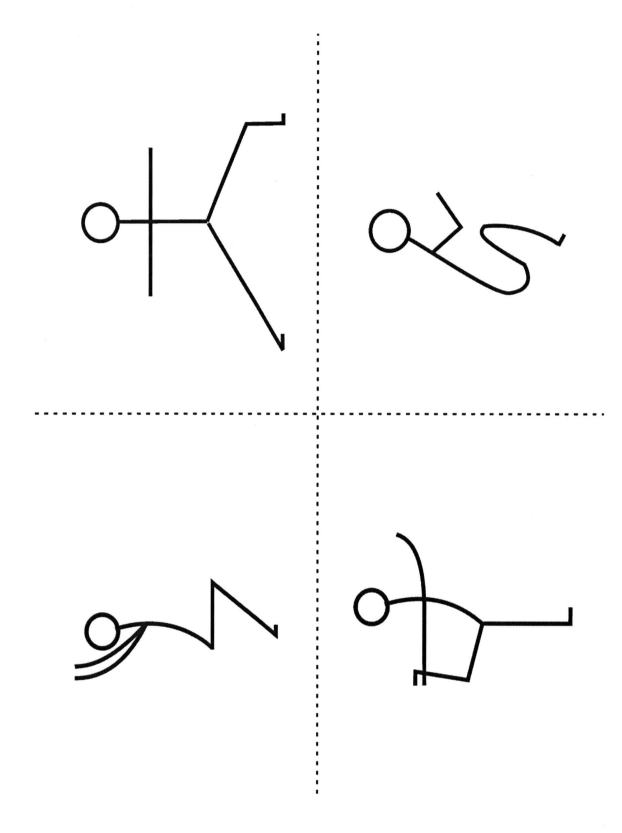

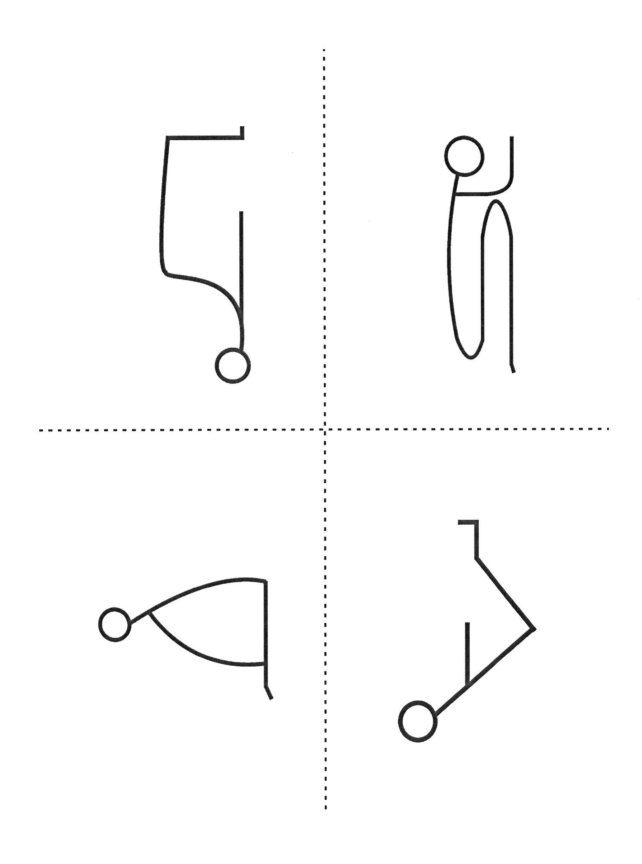

April Merrilee

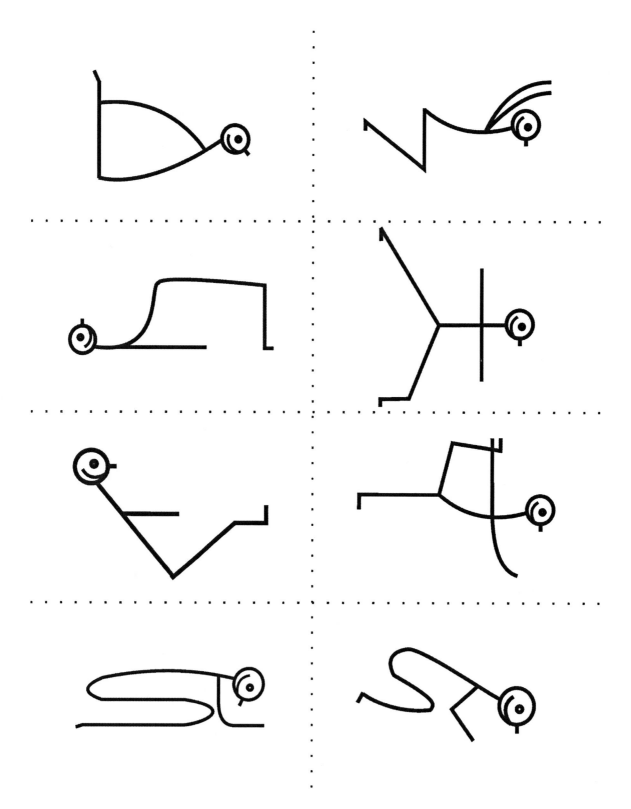

possum	rain
pig	wind
farmer	crow
pumpkin	turkey

Basic Sentence Worksheet   The Magic Garden

Copy these sentences next to the correct drawing on the following page.

The rain is wet.

The wind is cold.

The crow can fly.

The turkey is brown.

The possum is sleeping.

The pig is so big.

The farmer is nice.

The pumpkin is orange.

Challenge Sentence Worksheet: Match and copy next to the correct drawing!

I have a very good tractor.

I can make funny noises with my throat.

I make the leaves fly all around.

I like to nap in a tree.

I am black and very loud.

I water all the vegetables.

I am tasty inside a pie!

I love to roll around in the mud.

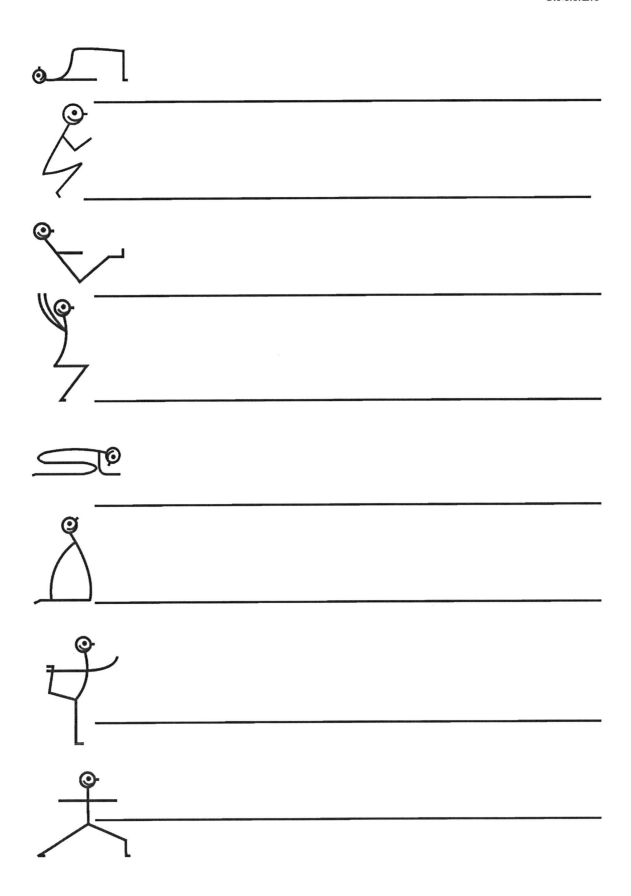

April Merrilee

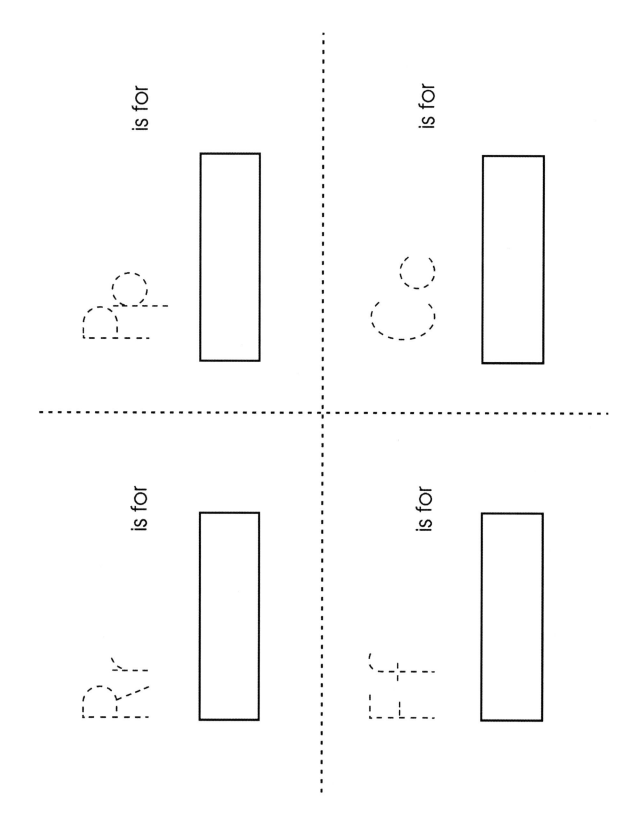

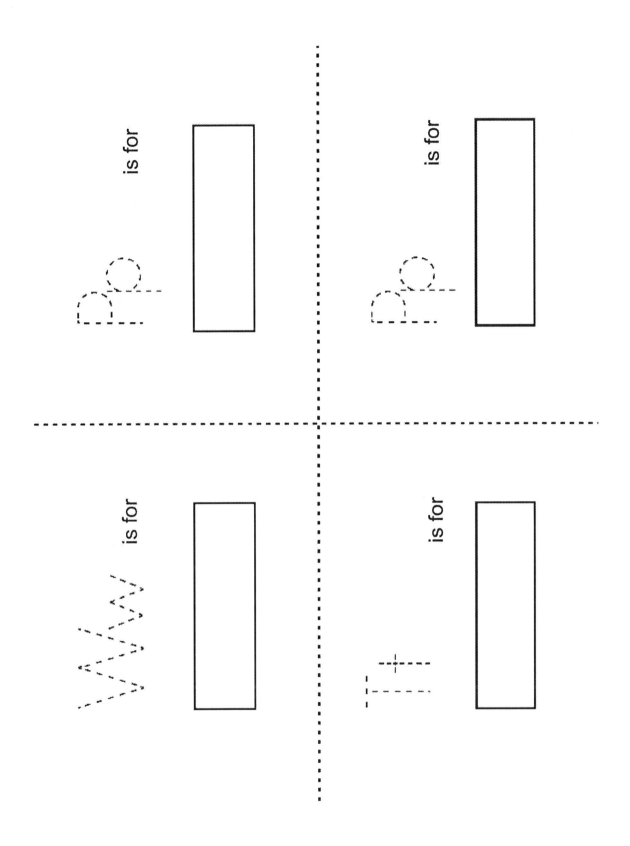

ROUTINE # 2: TOM CAT

Tom cat lives at the edge of a big forest. He has a favorite pine tree that is so very, very tall! From the top of his favorite tree, he can look out from the forest across the meadow, over the river to the mountains in the distance. He loves to climb to the very tip top and watch all the animals coming and going in and out of the forest, playing in the meadow and drinking from the river. Sometimes, Tom's animal friends come up the tree to visit with Tom. They each have their own way of getting up to the tip top. The falcon flies; the monkey swings; the panda climbs; the eagle soars; the cougar jumps; the turkey leaps; the peacock hops; and the raccoon scurries. After visiting, when he's by himself, Tom takes a little cat nap in his tree, curled up beside the tree trunk on the very top branch of this great big old pine. Nothing like a good nap to help a cat feel his very best! Well, that is, the nap is nice, but waking up in the tip top of a tall tree is not always such a great thing. Usually, Tom gets scared when he wakes up way at the top, and suddenly finds that he is stuck. Can't move a muscle to get himself down!! When he's stuck like that, he's so afraid he's going to fall out of that tree, all the way down to the ground. That would be such a long fall!! So, he doesn't move. He has to wait for his animal friends to come along on their way in and out of the forest so he can ask for help. Sometimes, it's a very long wait while Tom wonders who will be the first to show up. Let's sing about old Tom waiting up there in the tree.

LANGUAGE HIGHLIGHTS

- /s/ blends
- Initial /f/ sounds
- /r/ sounds
- Rhyming words
- Synonyms for common verbs
- Alliteration
- Optional: Sign language for action words

April Merrilee

TOM CAT
Sung to the tune of "On Top of Old Smoky"
Intro (sing while standing and clapping hands or crossing midline):

On top of old pine tree
Oh, Tom he was stuck
He waited for his friends
To bring him some luck

Repeat intro between first and second verses

First verse:

He said I want **falcon**
To **fly** to the top
If he will come help me
I won't fall flip flop

He said I want **monkey**
To **swing** to the top
If he will come help me
I won't fall flip flop

He said I want **panda**
To **climb** to the top
(repeat above lines)

He said I want **eagle**
To **soar** to the top…..

He said I want **cougar**
To **jump** to the top…….

He said I want **turkey**
To **leap** to the top

He said I want **peacock**
To **hop** to the top

He said I want **raccoon**
To **scoot** to the top

Second verse:

He waited for **falcon**
To come help him down
But **falcon** did not **fly**
And Tom wears a frown

He waited for **monkey**
To come help him down
But **monkey** did not **swing**
And Tom wears a frown

He waited for **panda** to come help him down
But **panda** did not **climb**
And Tom wears a frown

He waited for **eagle** to come help him down
But **eagle** did not **soar** ……..

He waited for **cougar** …………
But **cougar** did not **jump**………….

He waited for **turkey**…………
But **turkey** did not **leap**……………..

He waited for **peacock**……………
But **peacock** did not **hop**……………….

He waited for **raccoon** to come help him down
At last raccoon did scoot, Tom's back on the ground

Tom said I do thank you
My friend the raccoon
You're such a good helper
Bet I'll see you soon

Conclusion: Ask children if Tom got down. Why did Tom say he'd see the raccoon soon? (because he'll go back up and get stuck in the tree again).

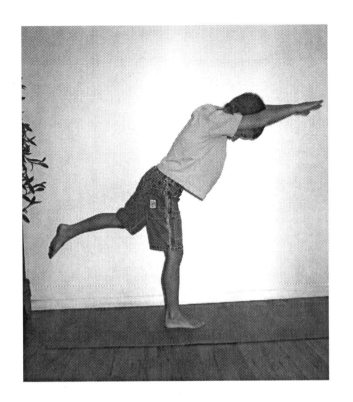
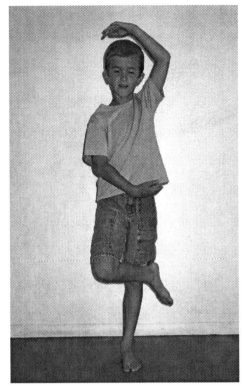
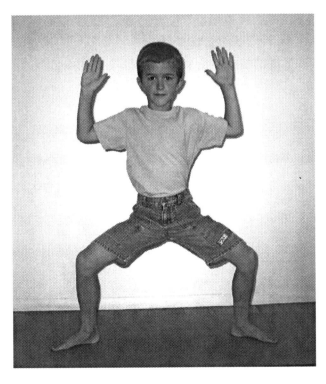
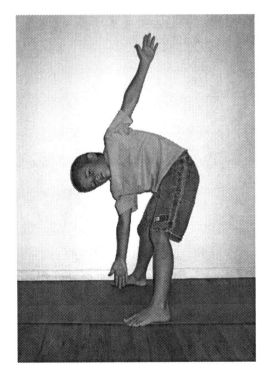

April Merrilee

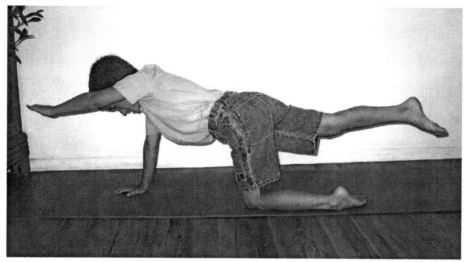
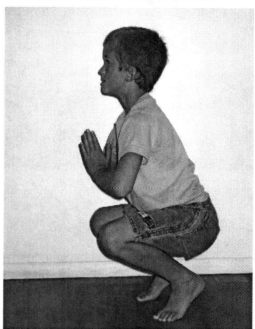
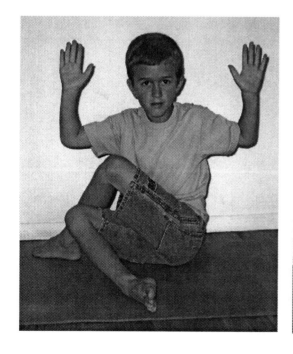
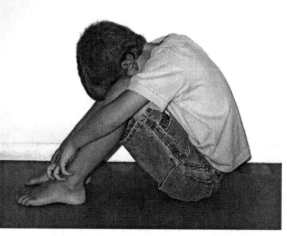

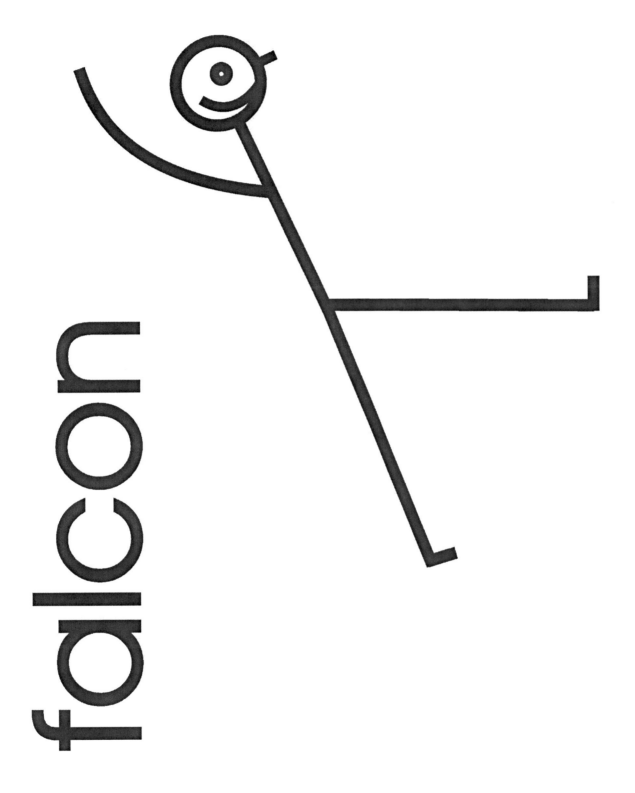

monkey

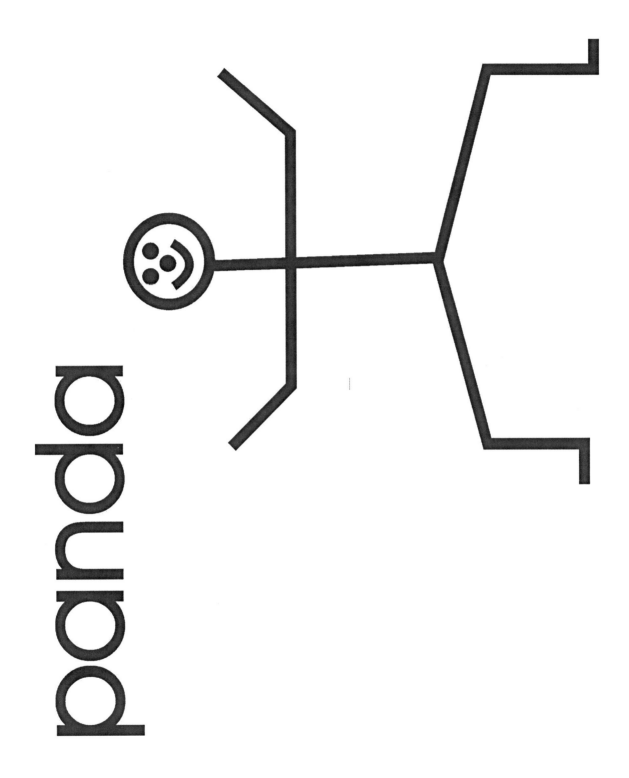

eagle

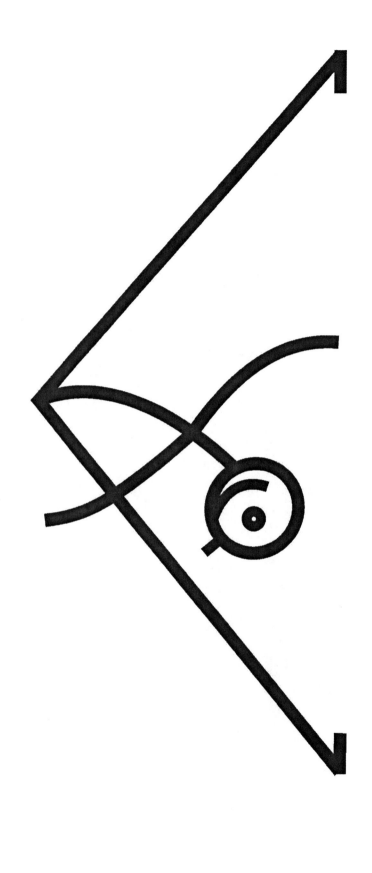

cougar

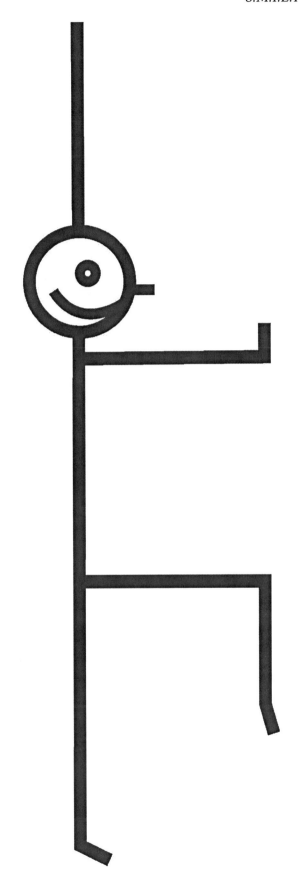

April Merrilee

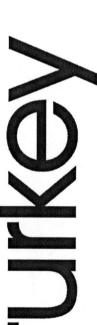

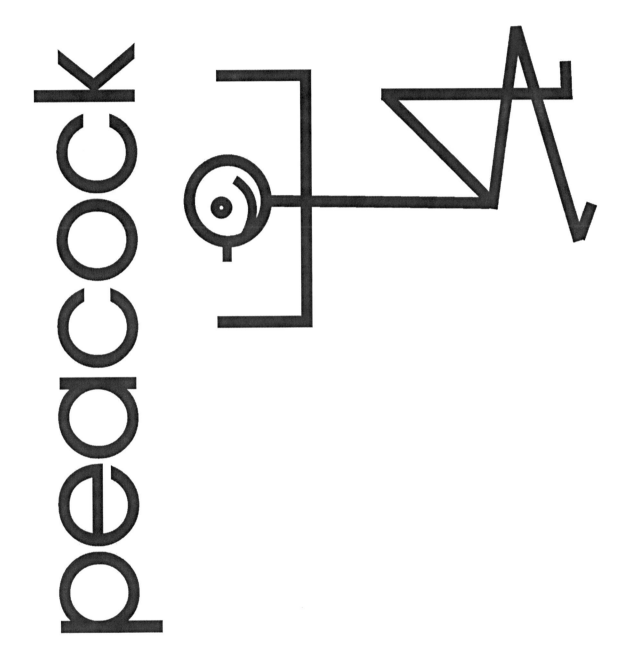

April Merrilee

racoon

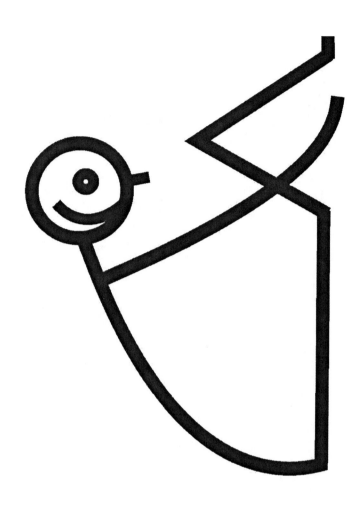

falcon

monkey

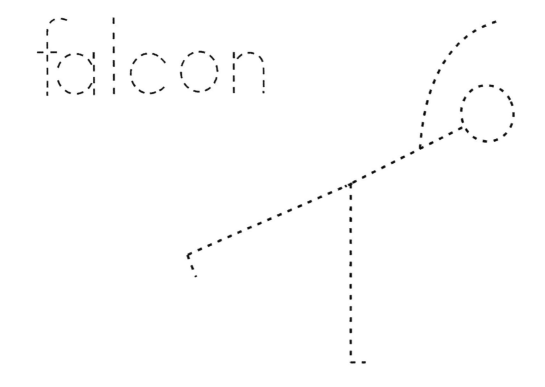

April Merrilee

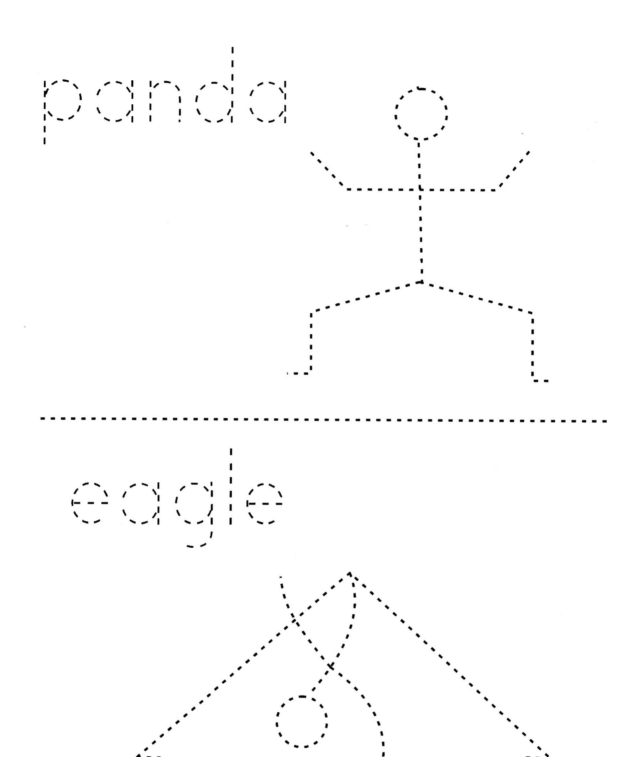

cougar

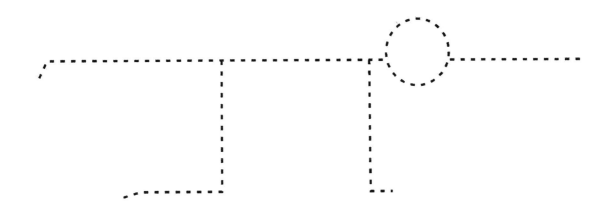

turkey

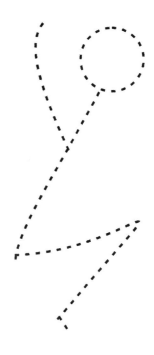

April Merrilee

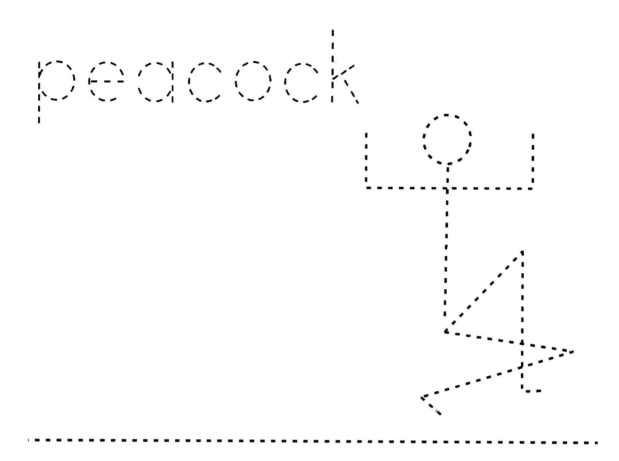

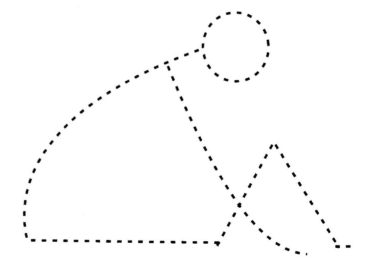

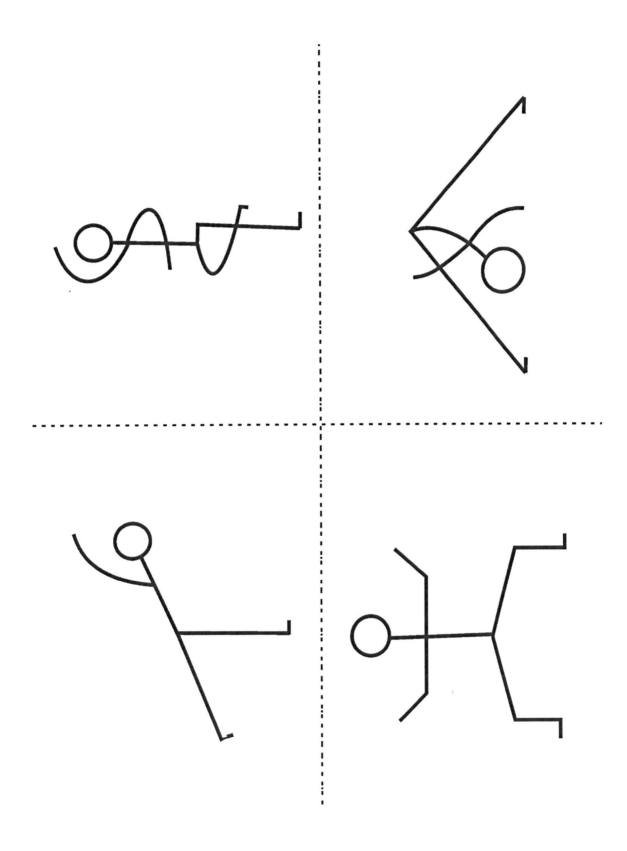

April Merrilee

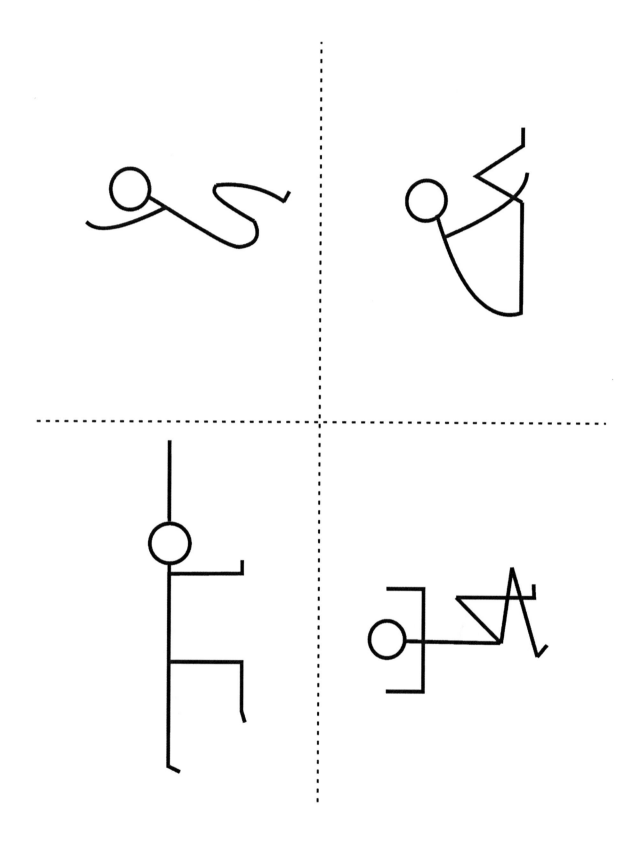

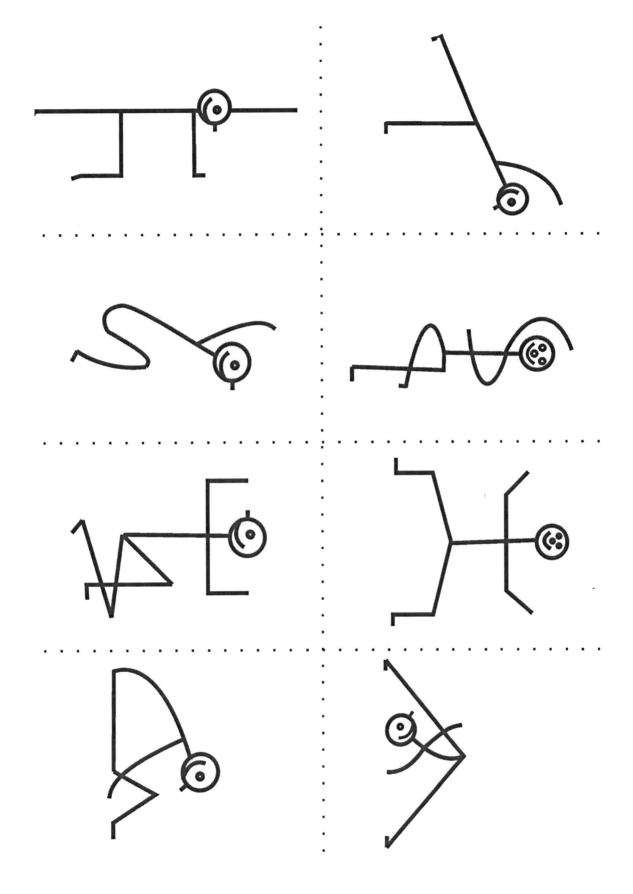

cougar	falcon
turkey	monkey
peacock	panda
racoon	eagle

Basic Sentence Worksheet   Tom Cat

Copy these sentences next to the correct drawing on the following page.

The falcon can fly.

The monkey is funny.

The panda is cute.

The eagle is a big bird.

The cougar is a fast cat.

A turkey can jump high.

The peacock is pretty.

The raccoon is shy.

Challenge Sentence Worksheet: Match and copy next to the correct drawing!

I am a very special bird.

I can fun fast like a lion.

I like to swing in the trees.

I have the most beautiful feathers.

I hunt small animals from the sky.

We have to hide from humans!

I wear a mask around my eyes.

I am really a small bear.

April Merrilee

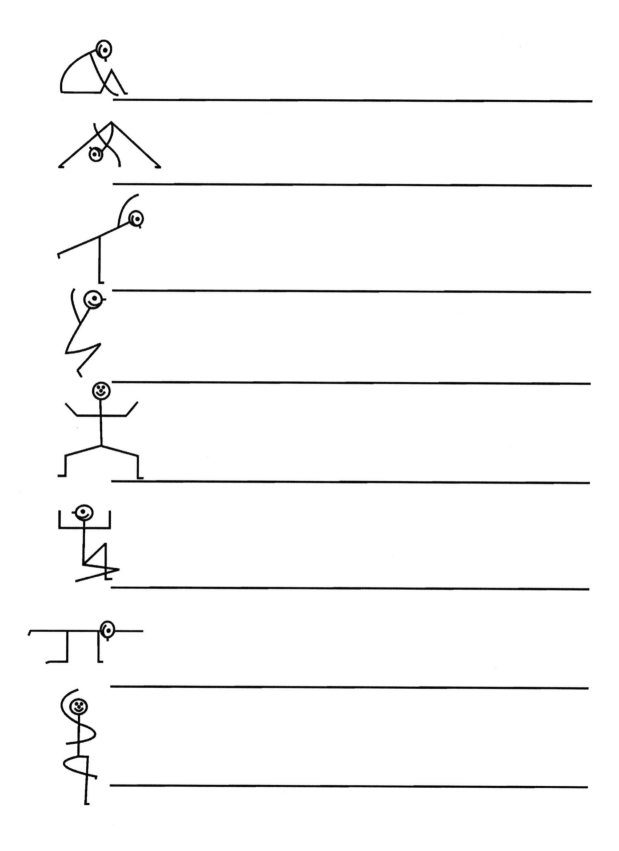

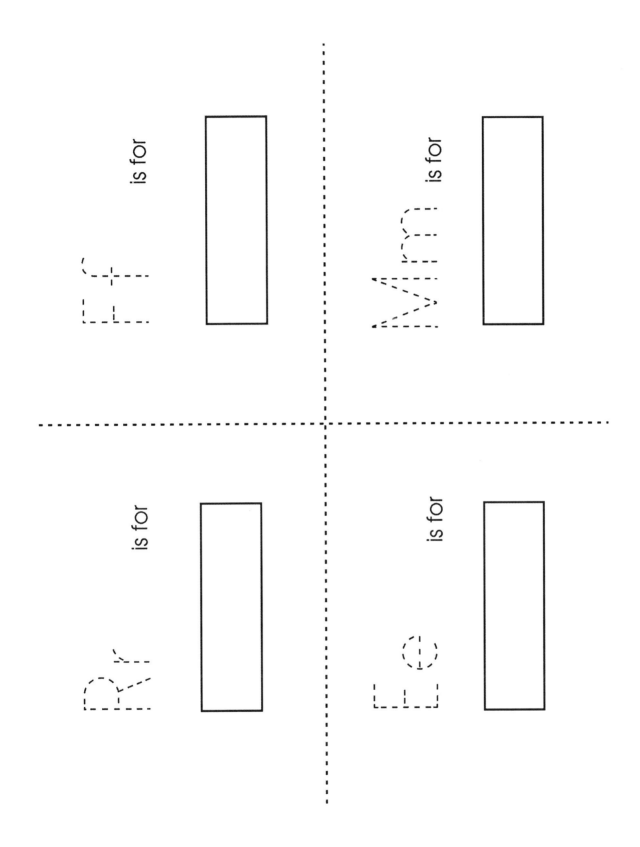

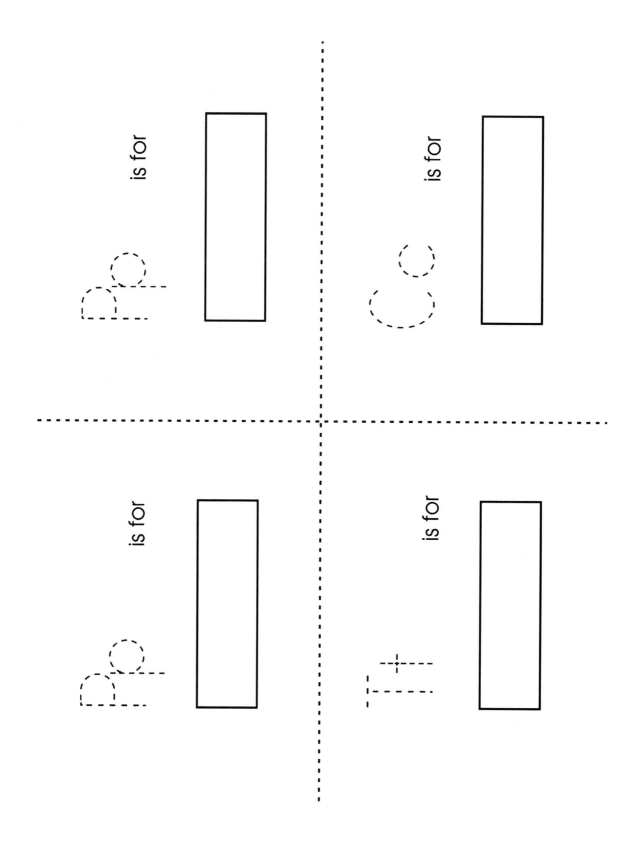

ROUTINE # 3: GUESS WHO

There was once a sweet old Lion who lived all alone in a cave. Sometimes he would come out of his cave and walk through the woods, visiting with all his animal friends. There came a time when the animals noticed that Lion was very grumpy.

Discussion: "What does grumpy mean? Do you ever get grumpy? I do!

"What are some other words for grumpy? What makes you feel grumpy?"

Teach sign language for mad and sad. Say those rhyming words.

"If somebody is grumpy, does that make them a bad person?"

"No, maybe they're just having a bad day"

"How do you think Lion's friends could tell he was grumpy?"

"What do you think made him feel grumpy?"

Lion's friends knew he was really grumpy because, while walking through the woods he would roar and roar, louder and louder. This was very unlike Lion, because usually he was just fine and happy living in his cave and talking his walks.

Let me hear you roar like a lion !! 3 times, then use sign language for STOP).

Lion's friends decided they wanted to do something to help cheer him up.

"**If you wanted to cheer up a friend who was feeling bad, what would you do?**"

(take turns with children sharing their ideas)

Well, Lion's friends wanted to play a fun guessing game with him. They decided to send him secret notes. "**Do you know what made the notes secret?**"

They were secret because nobody put their names on their notes. So Lion had to guess who sent each one. The animals made it a little easier on him by giving him a clue. "**What's a clue?**" (or a hint)

Well, here's what the animals did. Each one of them drew a picture on their note of something that rhymes with the animal's name. That way, if Lion could figure out the rhymes, then he might guess who sent the notes.

Optional: Introduce what each animal drew (see song lyrics). Can ask children: "What rhymes with stork, what picture would a stork draw?.... "What's a word that sounds like crow, what would a crow draw?" etc., etc.

LANGUAGE HIGHLIGHTS

- Rhyming words
- Vocabulary: words for emotions
- Sign language for emotions
- Grammar: forming questions
- Synonyms (smile/grin; hint/clue)
- Final /g/ sound
- /sh/ sound

GUESS WHO
Sung to the tune of "Home on the Range"

Intro (chorus melody - sing while standing and clapping/crossing midline)

Oh, who wrote the note
That made the Lion smile
Each one had a clue
Saying, "Can you guess who"
Lion thought really hard for a while

Repeat chorus between verses

First verse (stanza melody):

It could be the **stork**
Would a **stork** draw a **fork**?
Do you think
As a clue that would work?

It could be the **crow**
Would a **crow** draw a **bow**?
Do you think
That would help Lion know?

(insert names of animals & objects)
Fish…….dish
Do you think that would be the best wish?

Cat………..hat
Do you think Lion would guess from that?

Dog…….log
Do you think that would clear up the fog?

Bug………jug
Do you think that's as good as a hug?

Pig……..wig
Do you think as a clue that's so big?

Hare………chair
Do you think Lion knows his friends care?

Second verse (stanza melody)

So he told the **stork**
Your clue **really did work**
I can grin
With my friend and his **fork**

So he told the **crow**
Your clue **did help me know**
I can grin
With my friend and his **bow**

(insert lines from above)
…**fish**, your clue was my best wish
I can grin with my friend and his **dish**

….**cat**, your clue made me guess that
I can grin with my friend and his **hat**

…**dog,** your clue did clear the fog
I can grin with my friend and his **log**

…**bug,** your clue is good as a hug
I can grin with my friend and his **jug**

…**pig,** your clue really was big
I can grin with my friend and his **wig**

…**hare**, your clue tells me you care
..grin with my friend and his **chair**

Conclusion: Ask children if Lion liked the guessing game, and which note was the one to make him smile or which picture was the best clue/hint.

April Merrilee

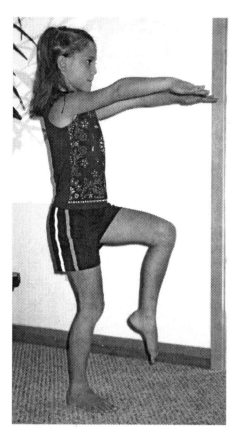
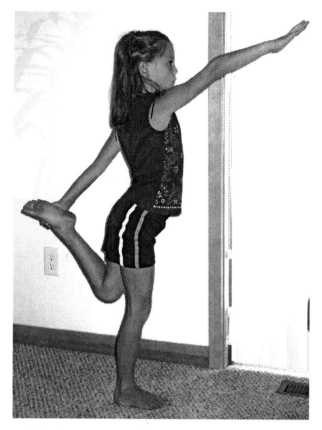
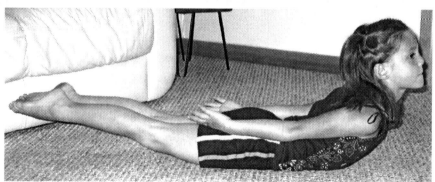
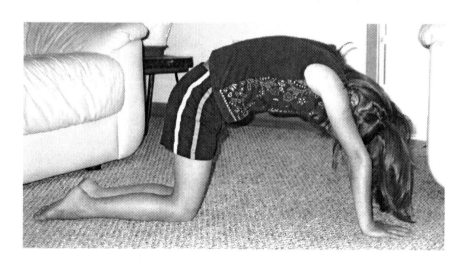

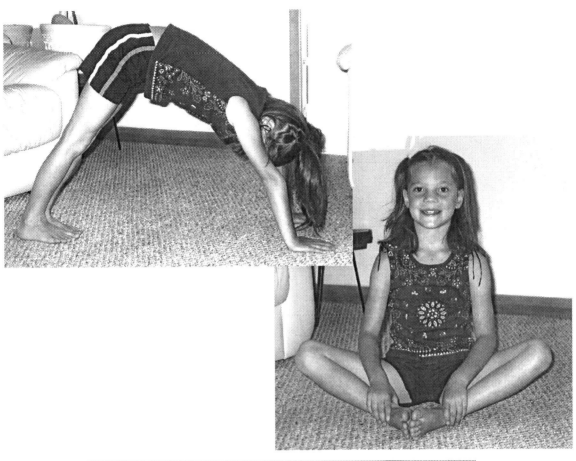
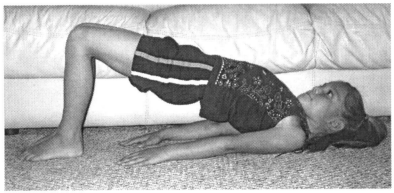
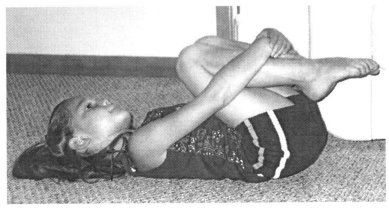

April Merrilee

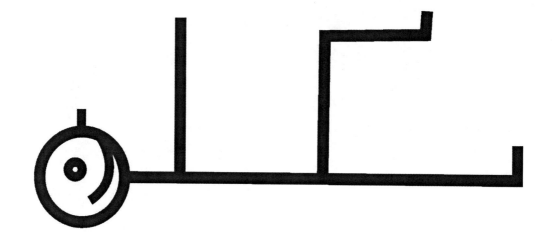

stork

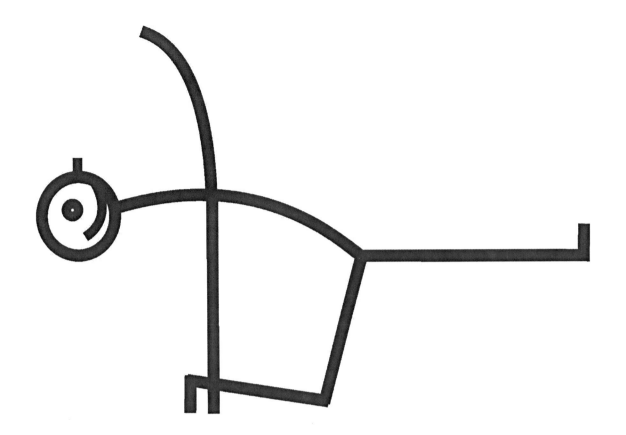

crow

April Merrilee

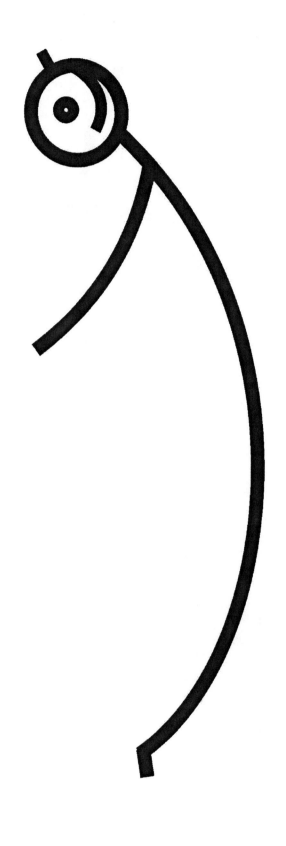

fish

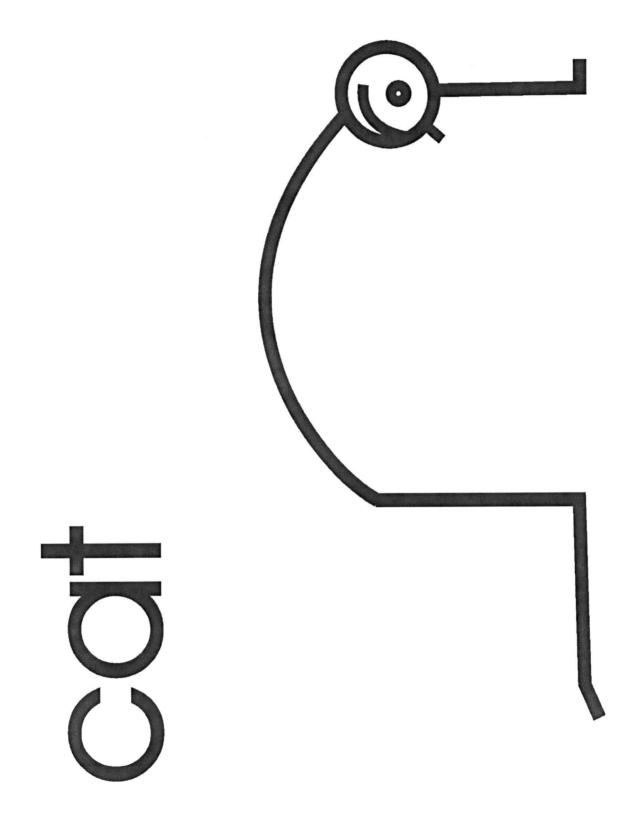

April Merrilee

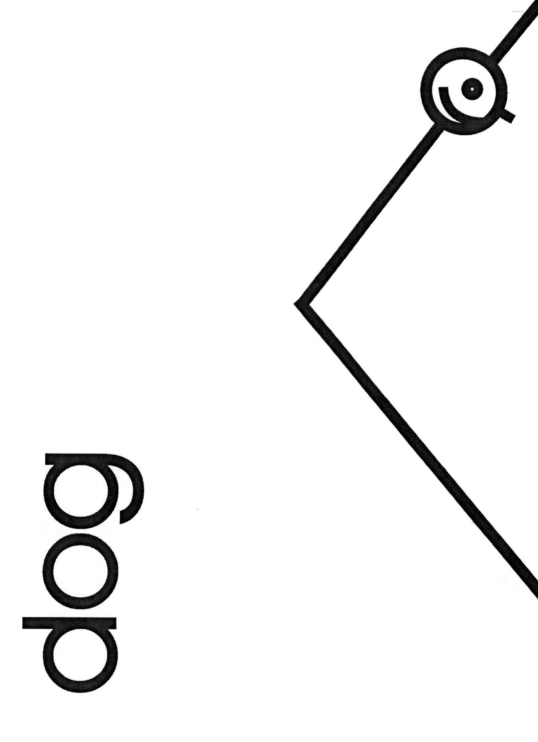

dog

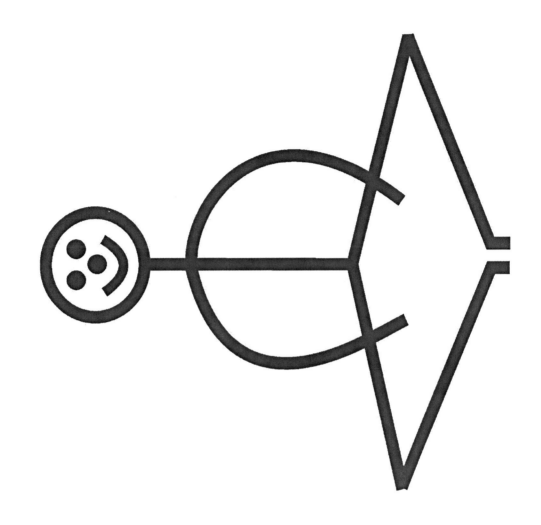

bug

April Merrilee

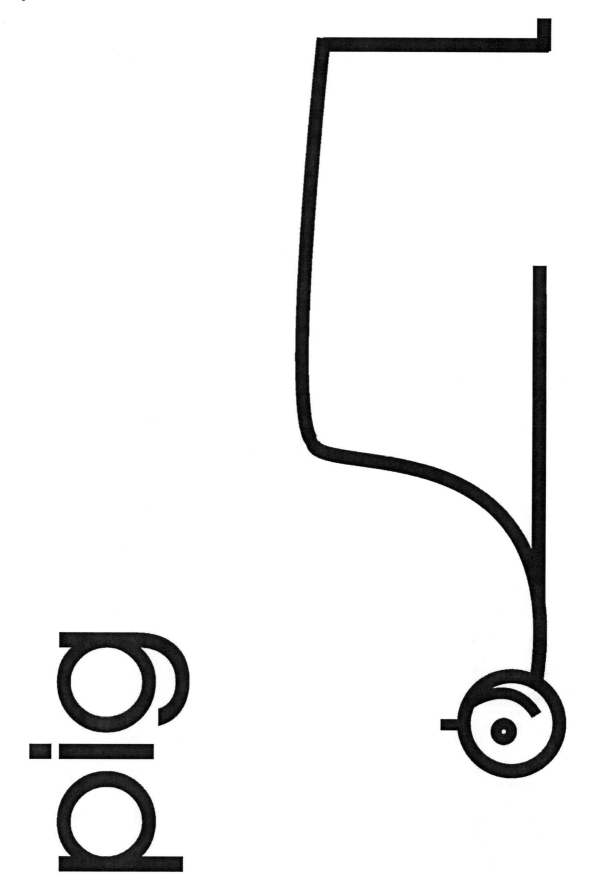

S.M.I.L.Y

hare

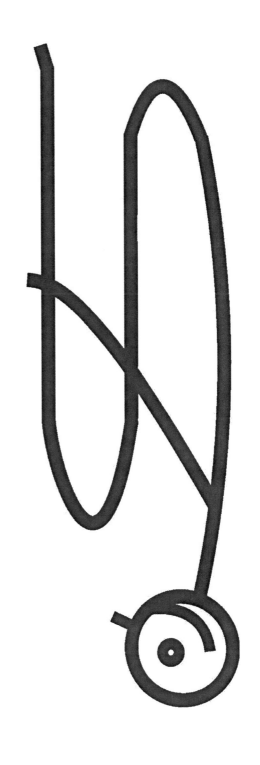

stork

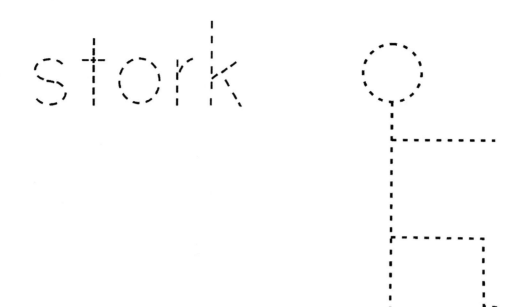

crow

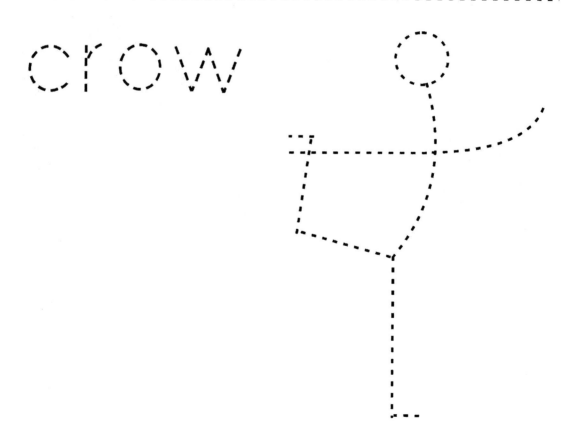

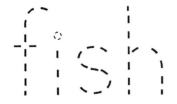

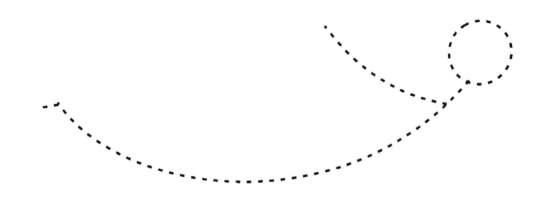

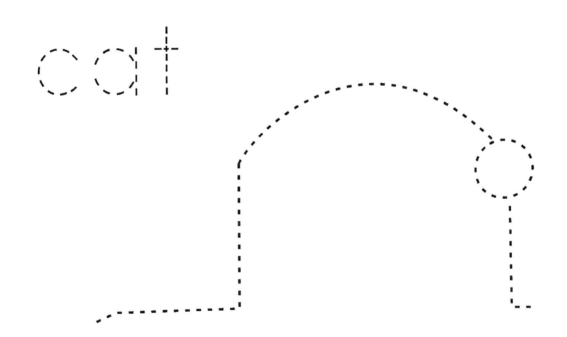

April Merrilee

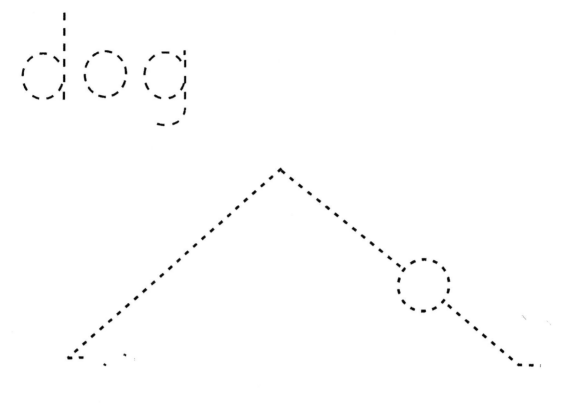

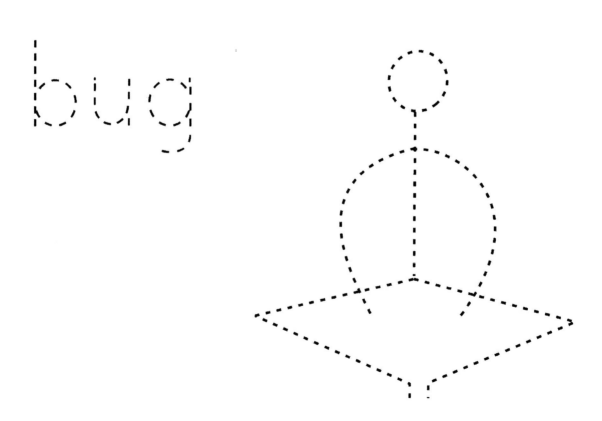

pig

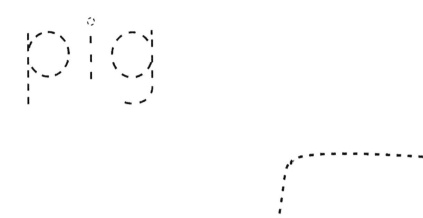

---

hare

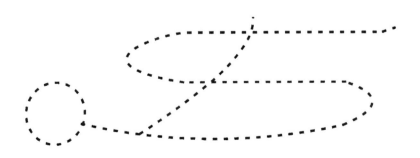

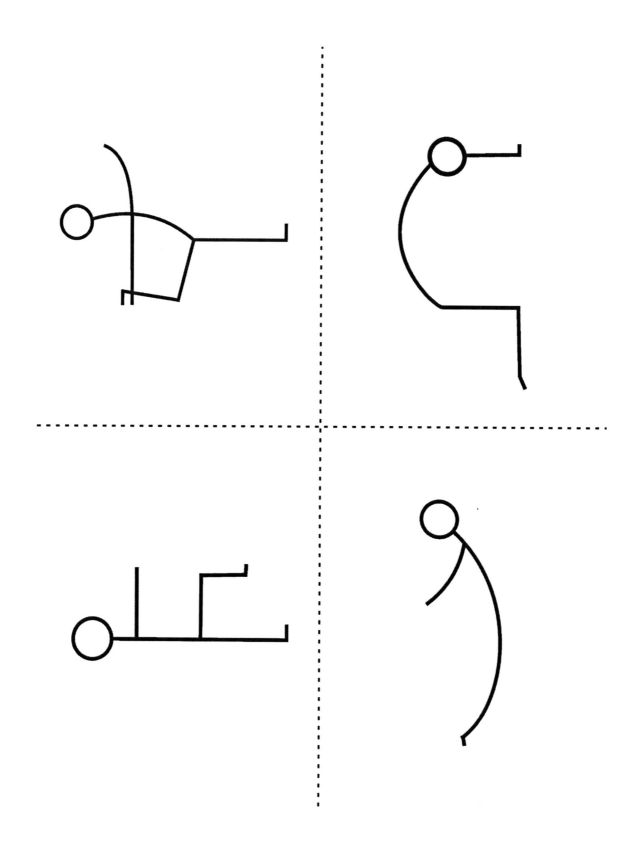

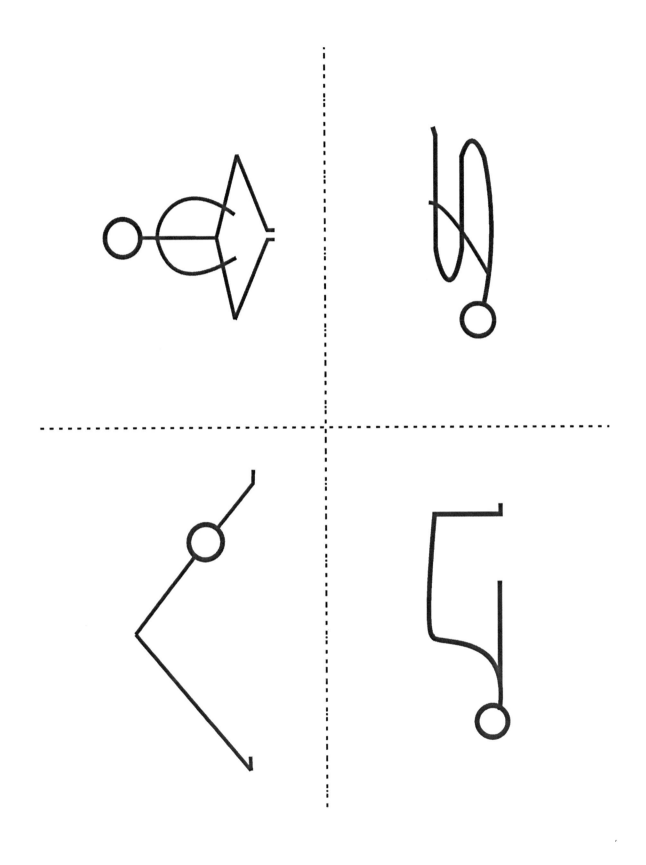

April Merrilee

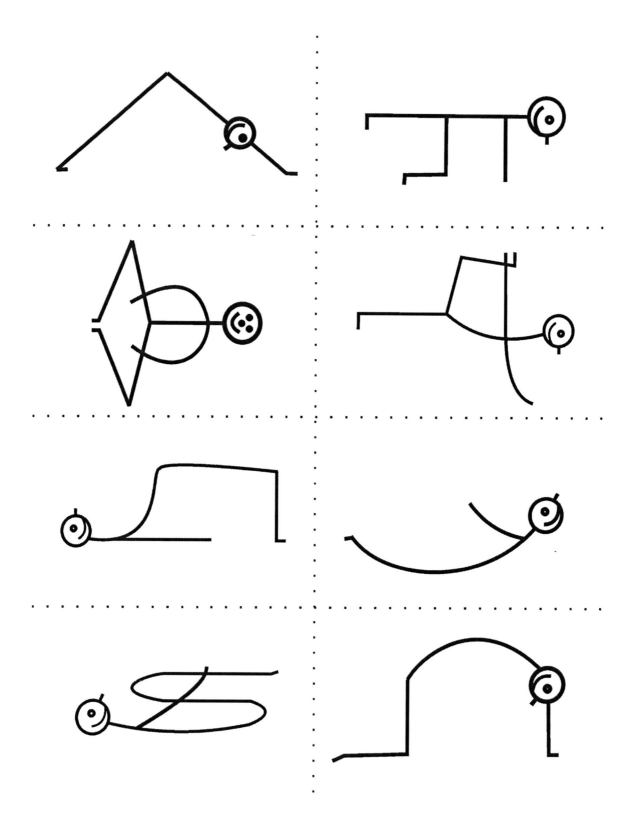

dog	stork
bug	crow
pig	fish
hare	cat

April Merrilee

Basic Sentence Worksheet   Guess Who

Copy these sentences next to the correct drawing on the following page.

The stork is a tall bird.

The crow is very black.

A fish can swim.

The cat likes to play.

The dog likes to run.

The bug is very small.

The pig is pink.

A hare is a bunny.

Challenge Sentence Worksheet: Match and copy to the correct drawing!

I am bigger than most rabbits.

I make a buzzing noise.

I live in the river or the lake.

I like to bury bones.

I have a very big beak.

I have a little curly tail.

I love to sleep in the sun.

My feathers are black and shiny.

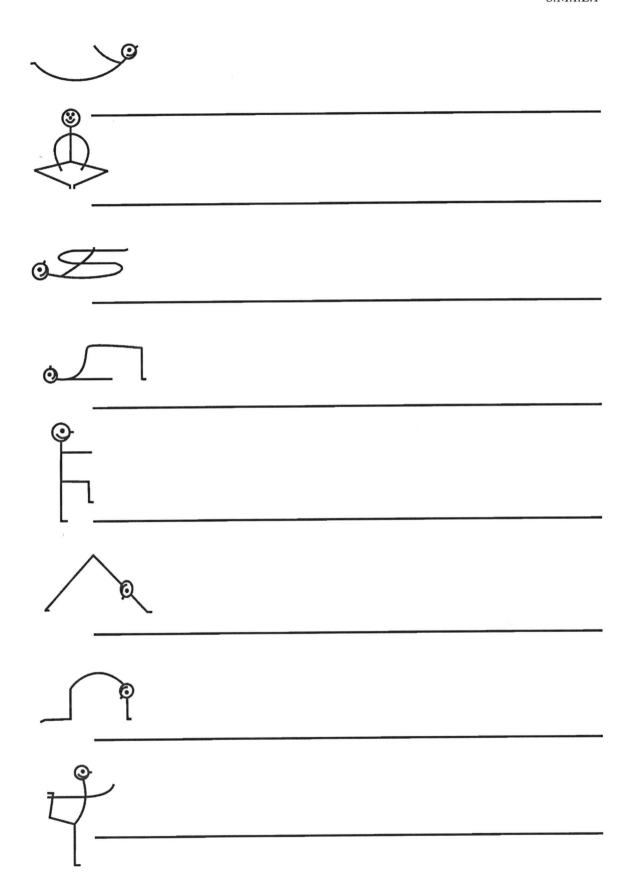

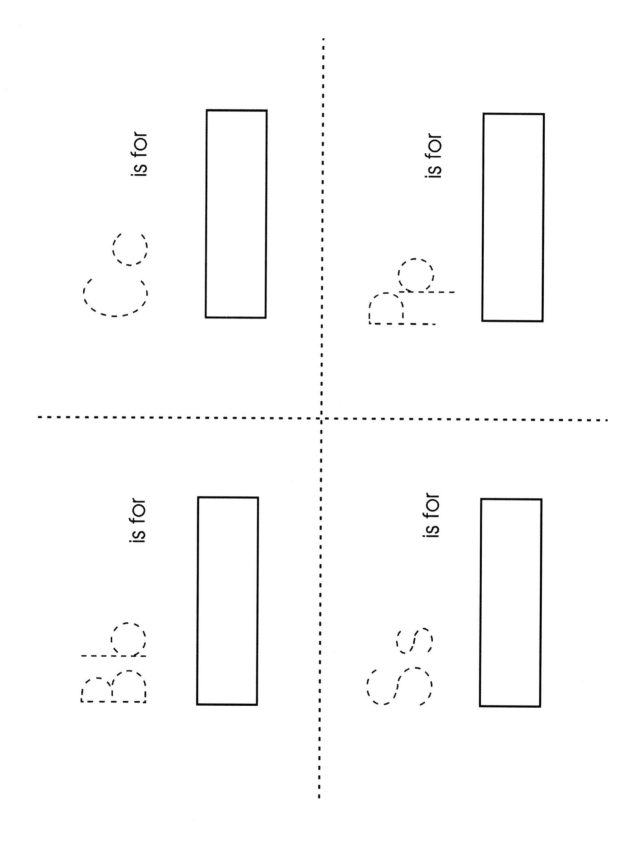

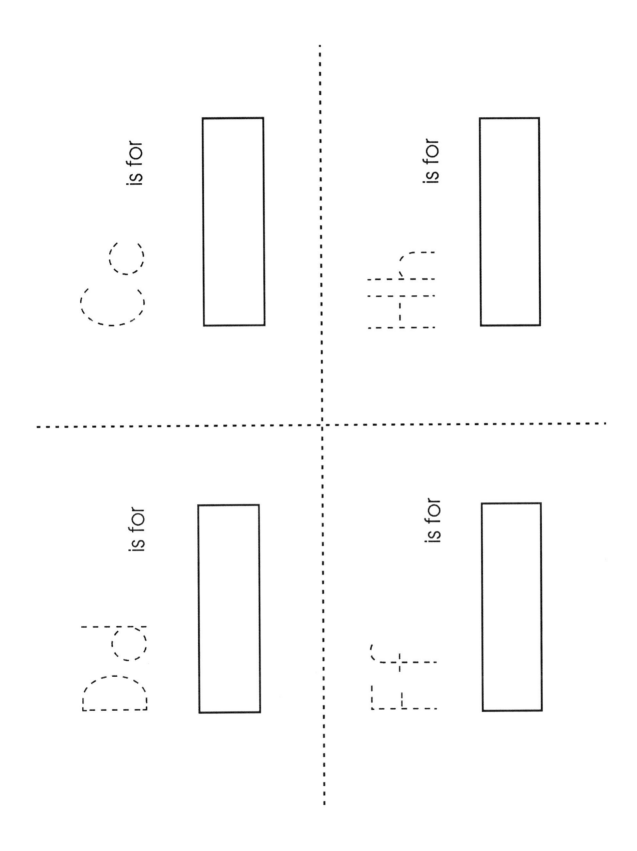

ROUTINE # 4: OLD MAN WINTER

This is a story about life and the seasons of the year. "Oooohhh, brrrrr!" (act cold) Why does a person say that, "oooohhh, brrrrr!" That's right, because they're cold. This time of year, it is cold outside and in some places it is snowing. Maybe the wind blows and the trees freeze! When it turns cold like this, we say it is winter. This is when people and animals like to be quiet and rest in the shelter of their homes. After winter, when it starts getting warmer, the plants grow and the flowers bloom. Then we say it is spring. After spring, the weather gets hot and the sun stays up for a long time after dinner. This is summer. We like summer to last a long time because it is so much fun. But after a while, the weather starts to cool down and we say it is fall or autumn. In the fall, the leaves on the trees change and make lots of beautiful, colorful patterns for us to enjoy. Then, it gets cold again and we're back to winter! So, we have spring, summer, fall and winter just like that. Did you know that these changes happen in people's lives, too? When we are babies, we are like the plants and flowers, growing and blooming. Babies are like spring time. Older children, like you, are like summer time – lots of long, fun days! Some of us want to stay like children forever. Grown ups are like fall, changing a lot and bringing many beautiful things into the world. And old people, especially very old people, are like winter. They are more quiet, and like to stay inside and rest. This is also a very special time of life, and can be a wonderful time of year, too. We even have the perfect nickname, for it: Old Man Winter. Old Man Winter is like the grandpa who brings us special surprises and lets us do extra fun stuff. Here is a song about all the fun things kids can do when Old Man Winter pays a visit.

Conclusion after singing: Ask children what would be the most fun of all the things we can do when Old Man Winter pays a visit.

LANGUAGE HIGHLIGHTS

- Verb tense changes: future perfect and past tense
- Irregular verbs (hear/heard; build/built; sit/sat; light/lit)
- Vocabulary: seasons of the year
- Metaphor (stages of life)
- Initial /w/
- Final /t/
- /s/ blends
- /l/ sound

OLD MAN WINTER - Sung to the tune of "London Bridge"

Old Man Winter's on his way
On his way, on his way
Old Man Winter's on his way
How will we play?

We will stomp in the **snow**
In the snow, in the snow
We will stomp in the snow
We'll say, "let's go"!

We will whisper in the **trees**
In the trees, in the trees
We will whisper in the trees
Maybe we'll freeze!

We will hear blowing **wind**
Blowing wind, blowing wind
We will hear blowing wind
Winter's our friend!

We will make our **snowman** tall
Snowman tall, snowman tall
We will make our snowman tall
And that's not all!

We will **skate** on the ice
On the ice, on the ice
We will skate on the ice
It looks so nice!

We will sing around the **fire**
'Round the fire, 'round the fire
We will sing around the fire
Come join our choir!

We will light a **candle** bright
Candle bright, candle bright
We will light a candle bright
Our favorite sight!

We will **sled** down the hill
Down the hill, down the hill
We will sled down the hill
What a great thrill!

Old Man Winter passed away
Passed away, passed away
Old Man Winter passed away
How did we play?

We stomped in the snow
In the snow, in the snow
We stomped in the snow
We said, "let's go"!

We whispered in the trees
In the trees, in the trees
We whispered in the trees
We did not freeze!

We heard blowing wind
Blowing wind, blowing wind
We heard blowing wind
Winter's our friend!

We made our snowman tall
Snowman tall, snowman tall
We made our snowman tall
And that's not all!

We skated on the ice
On the ice, on the ice
We skated on the ice
It was so nice!

We sang around the fire
'Round the fire, 'round the fire
We sang around the fire
Come join our choir!

We lit a candle bright
Candle bright, candle bright
We lit a candle bright
Our favorite sight!

We went sledding down the hill
Down the hill, down the hill
We went sledding down the hill
What a great thrill

April Merrilee

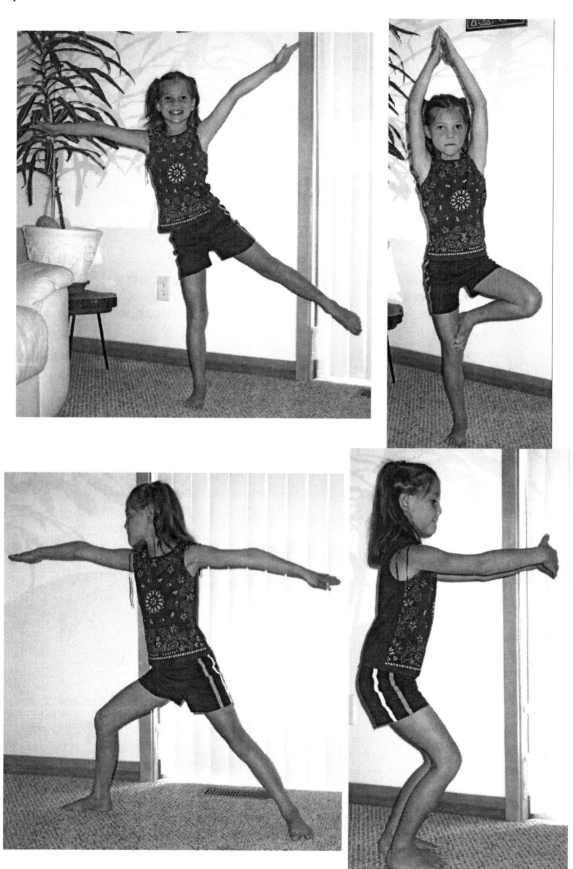

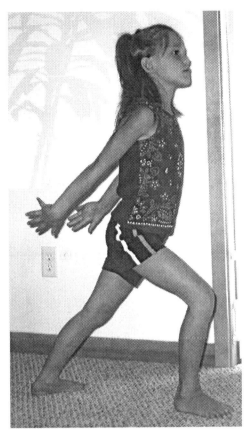
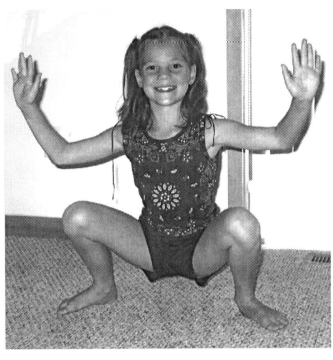
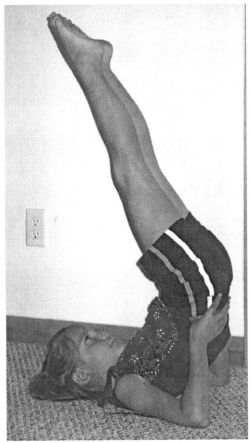
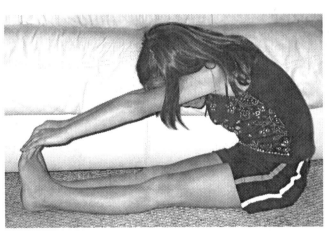

April Merrilee

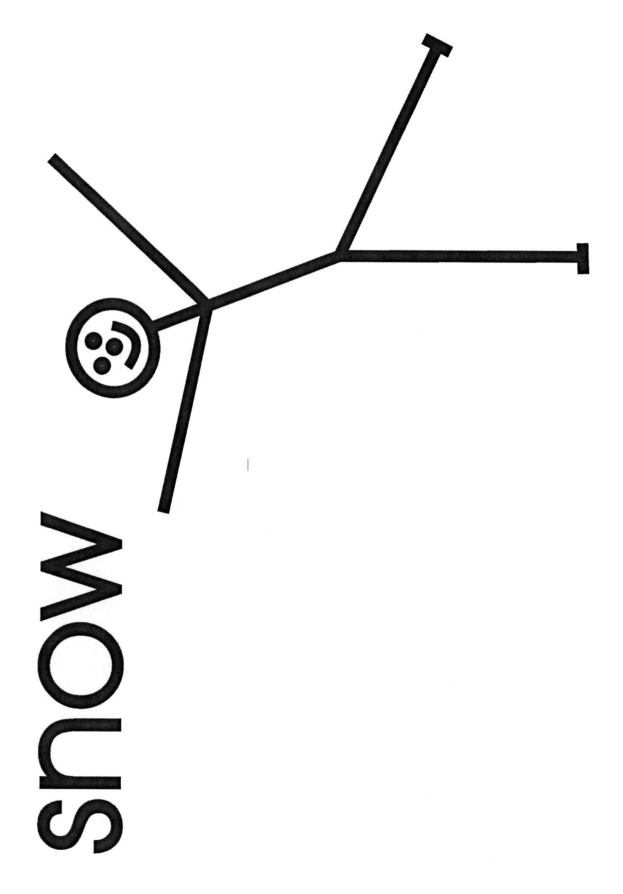

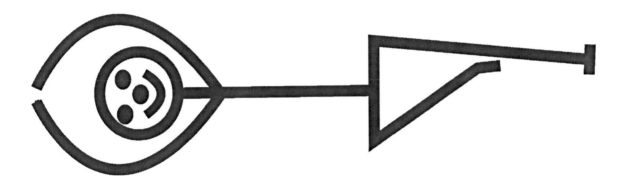

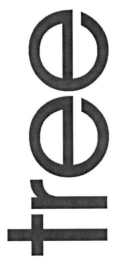

April Merrilee

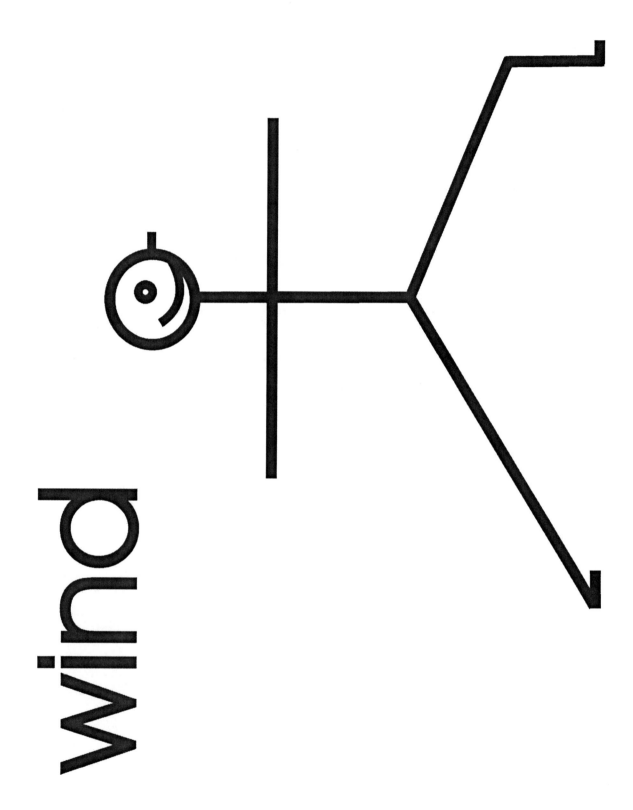

S.M.I.L.Y

snowmanonymous

April Merrilee

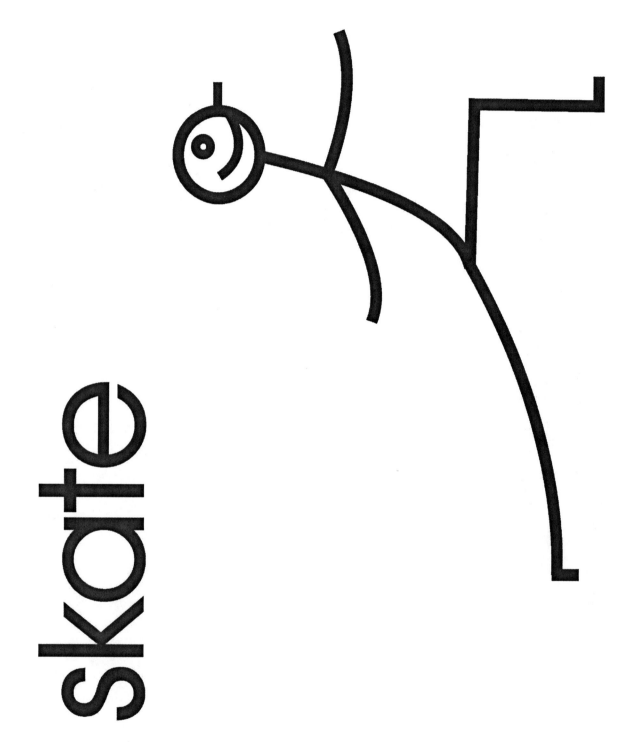

skate

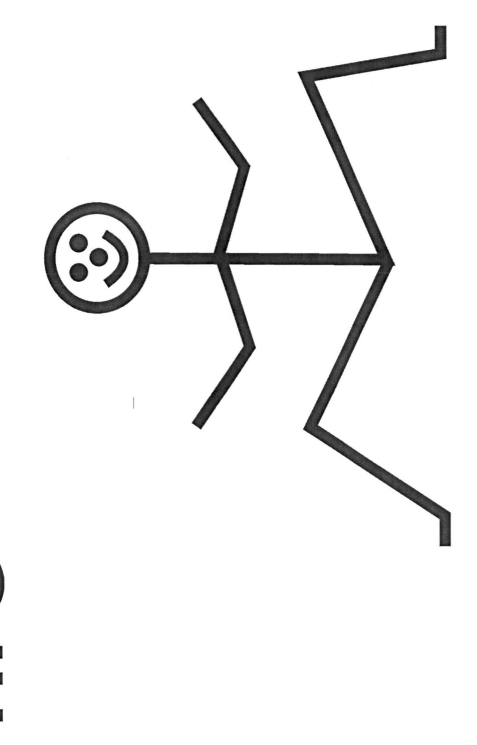

fire

April Merrilee

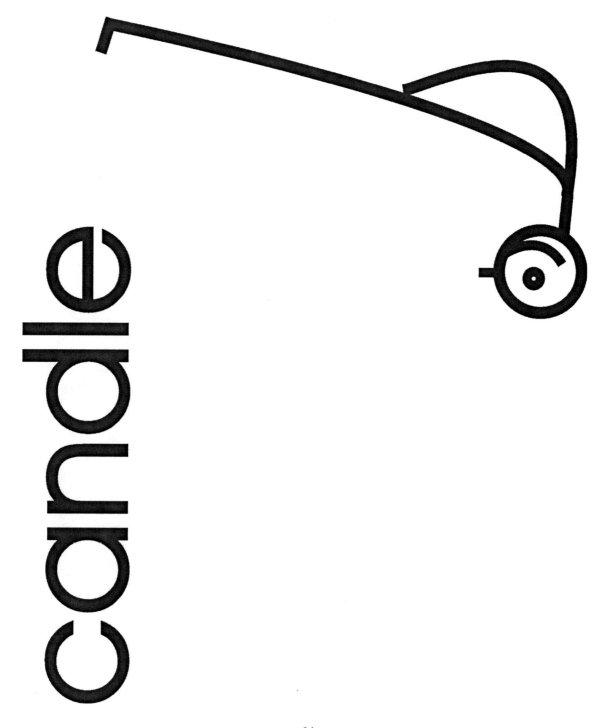

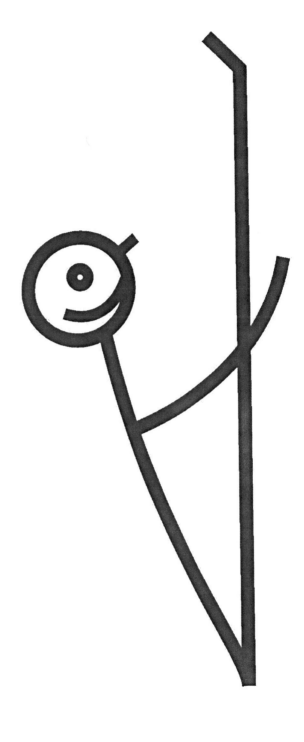

sled

April Merrilee

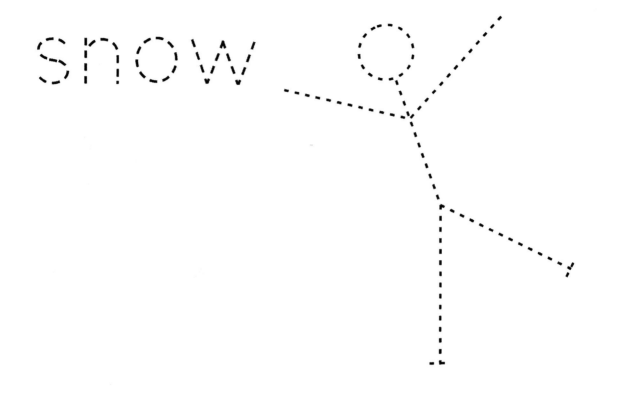

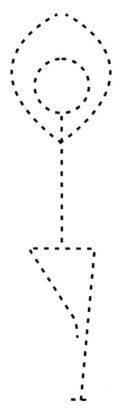

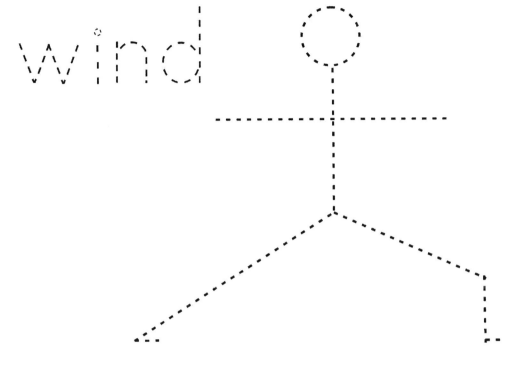
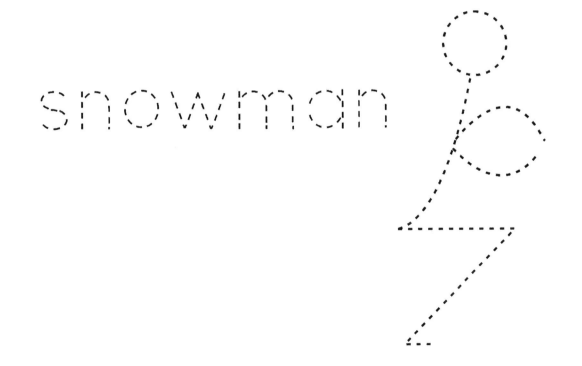

April Merrilee

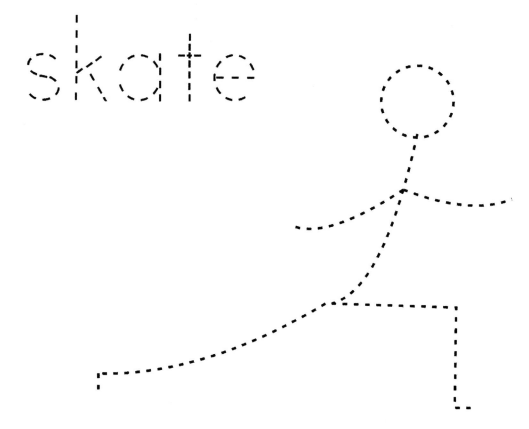

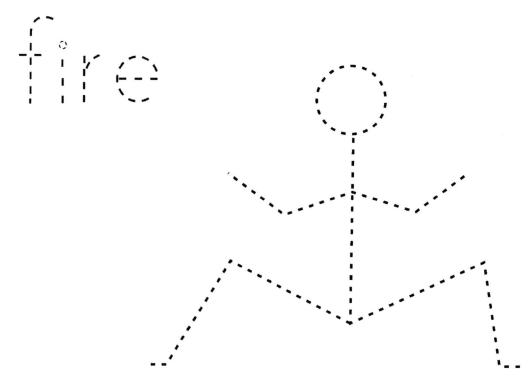

candle

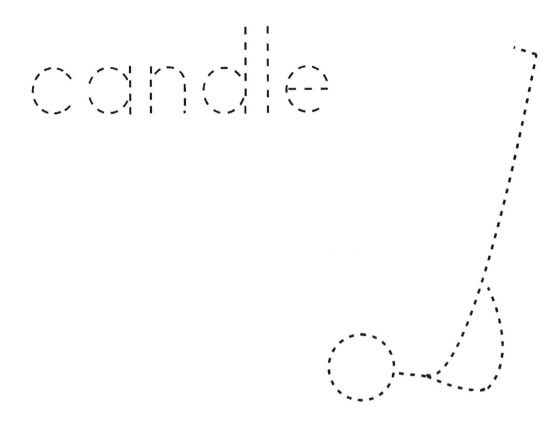

---

sled

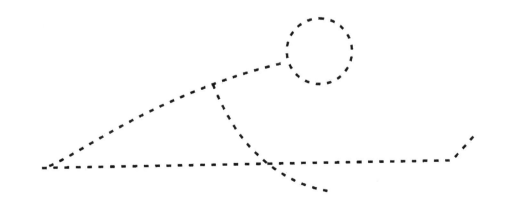

April Merrilee

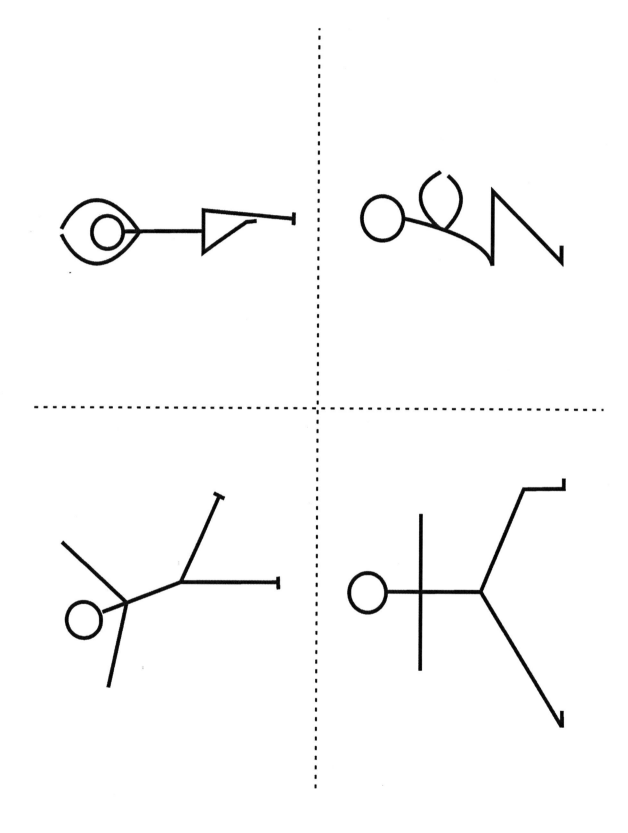

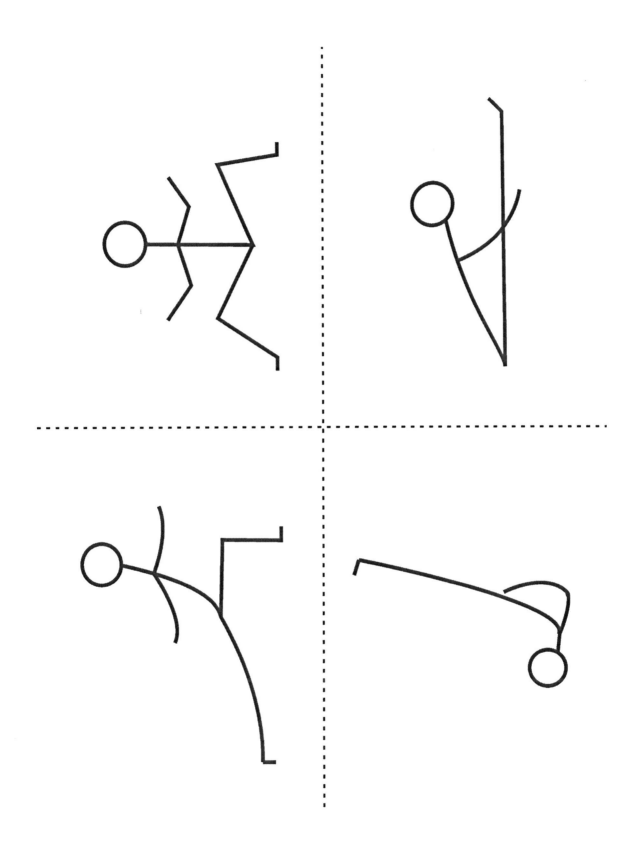

April Merrilee

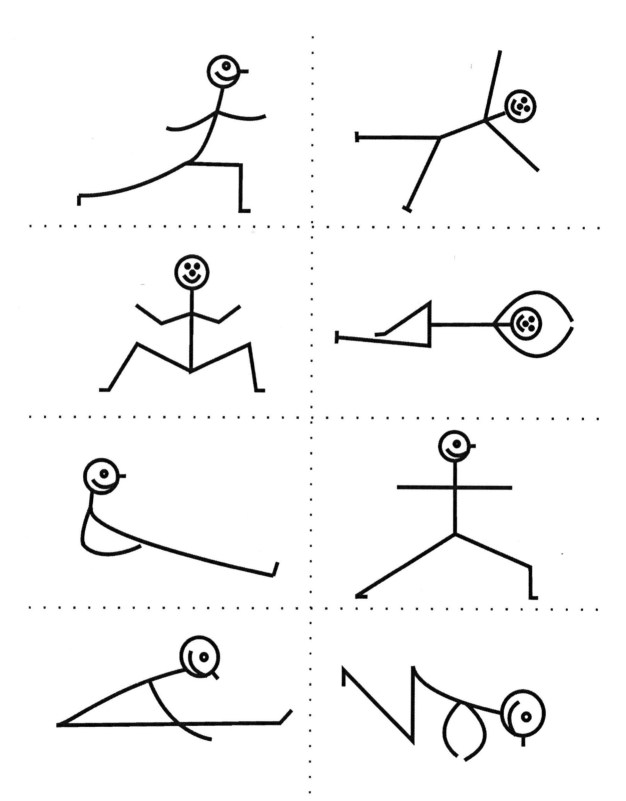

skate	snow
fire	tree
candle	wind
sled	snowman

Basic Sentence Worksheet Old Man Winter

Copy these sentences next to the correct drawing on the following page.

The snow is white.

A tree is tall.

The wind is cold.

My snowman looks good!

I like to skate.

The fire is warm.

Candles are so pretty.

My sled is fun.

Challenge Sentence Worksheet: Match and copy next to the correct drawing!

Let's go really fast down the hill!

I have a big round head.

Sometimes I come in a big storm.

I shine in a dark room.

This is fun all year long.

My roots go deep into the ground.

I can cook your food.

I howl through your windows.

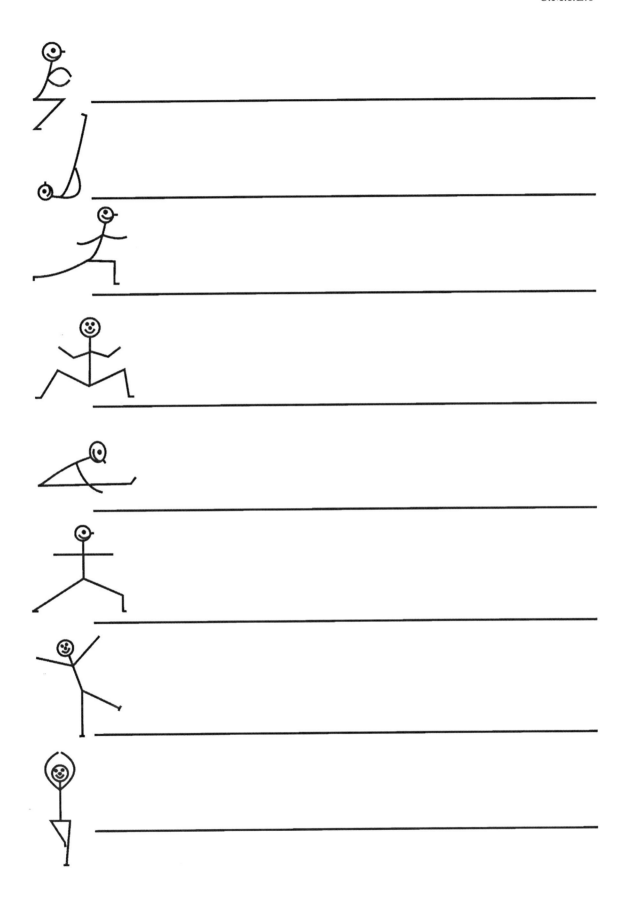

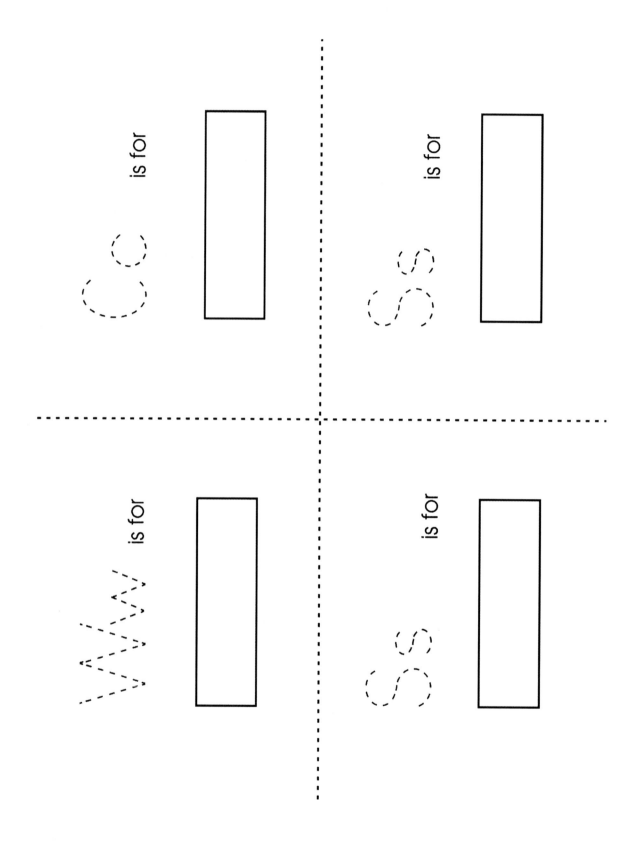

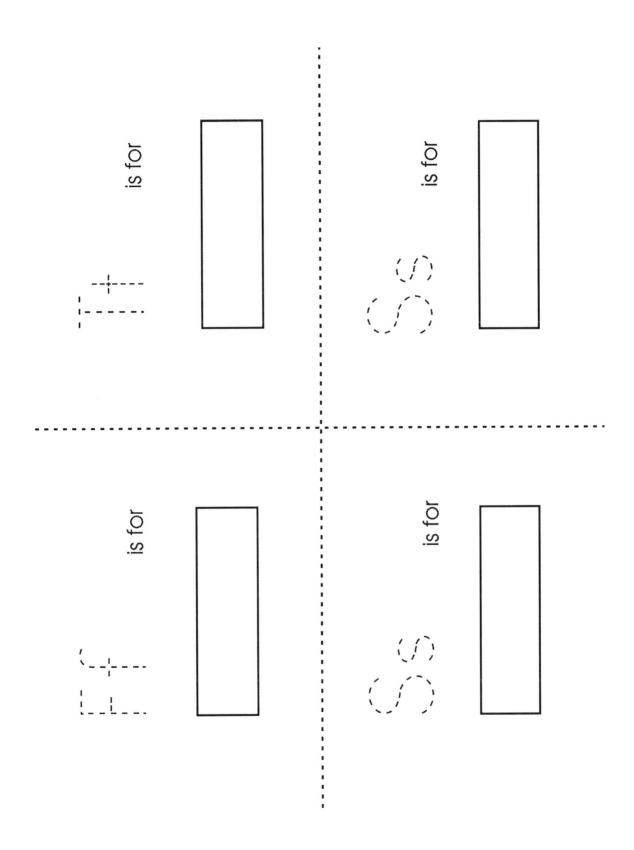

ROUTINE # 5: GOING ON SAFARI

There once was a young boy named Chaco, and his most favorite thing was to go to the zoo and watch all the animals. Have you ever been to the zoo? Which animals do you like best? Chaco especially liked watching the giraffes and the peacocks. He thought they were so lucky to have all those beautiful feathers. One day, Chaco got to meet the zookeeper while he was feeding the peacocks. Chaco told the zookeeper he thought the birds were the most beautiful animals in the zoo. The zookeeper said that the peacock knows how pretty those feathers are, and walks around all day strutting and saying, "I am sooooo beautiful!" (act like a strutting peacock). They were his favorite animal, too. Chaco also learned from the zookeeper that many of the animals were from a place far away called Africa - over on another continent! The zookeeper told Chaco that some people go all the way across the ocean to Africa on a special trip to see these animals living in their natural home. A journey like this to Africa is called a safari. Can you say that word? Safari. On a safari, people get to see lots of wild animals running free across the wide open African plains. They get to watch all sorts of exotic animals playing with each other, hunting their food, bathing in rivers, drinking from lakes and sleeping under bushes. When Chaco heard about going on safari, it was all he could think about. What an amazing thing to see! How he wanted to go on safari! He went home and told his parents all about the animals in Africa, and made up this song about what he wanted to do, so maybe his parents would take him.

Optional: Introduce animals (can print Google images, helpful with unfamiliar animal names) and their attributes within initial story. For example, "In Africa there is a bird called an ostrich. The ostrich thinks that when he puts his head in the ground, nobody can see him. He thinks he's hiding!" Or, "The flamingo is a pretty pink bird that can stand on one leg. Here's a picture of a standing flamingo", etc.

LANGUAGE HIGHLIGHTS

- Vocabulary: unfamiliar animals; Africa; safari
- Attributes: descriptive words for each animal
- Contractions: I'd; let's; we're; don't
- Initial /w/ sound
- Final /ing/ sound
- Initial /l/ sound
- /s/ blends

April Merrilee

GOING ON SAFARI
Sung to the tune of "Yankee Doodle"

First verse:	Second verse:
I want to go on safari Wonder what I'd see Maybe a **playing gorilla** What fun that would be!	Let's pretend we're on safari Oh, look right behind you I see a playing gorilla Don't you see it too?
I want to go on safari Wonder what I'd see Maybe a **stretching giraffe** What fun that would be!	Let's pretend we're on safari Oh, look right behind you I see a stretching giraffe Don't you see it too?

(repeat as above, insert animals)

Maybe a **standing flamingo**….	I see a **standing flamingo**…
Maybe a **hiding ostrich**….	I see a **hiding ostrich**…
Maybe a **hunting tiger**….	I see a **hunting tiger**…
Maybe a **swinging monkey**….	I see a **swinging monkey**…
Maybe a **strutting peacock**….	I see a **strutting peacock**…
Maybe a **sleeping 'gator**….	I see a **sleeping 'gator**…

Conclusion: Ask children, "Do you think his song got Chaco what he wanted? Do you think he got to go on safari with his parents? What would be the best thing about going on safari?"

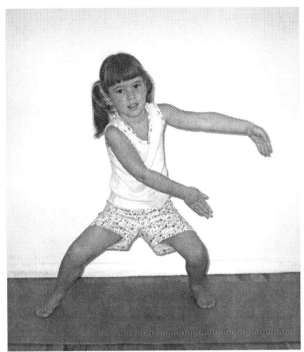
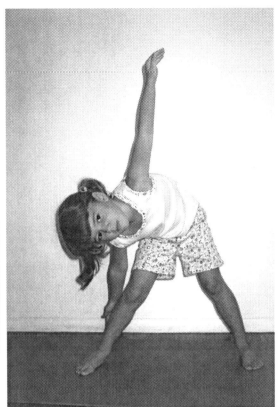
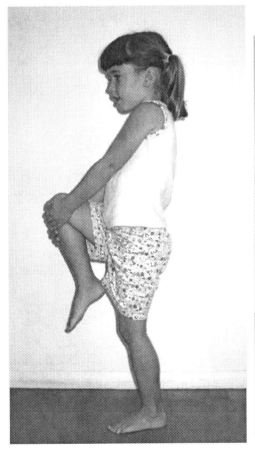
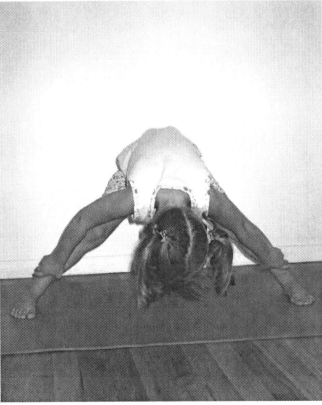

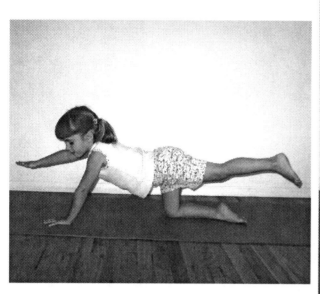
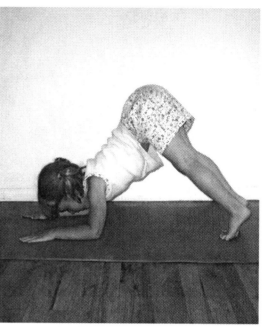
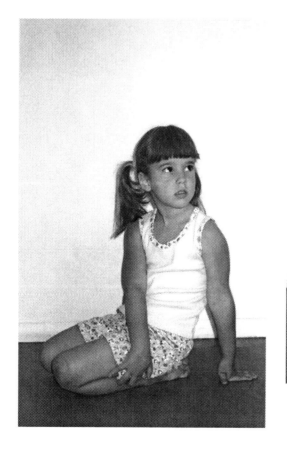
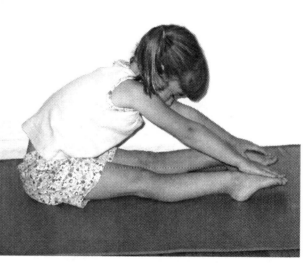

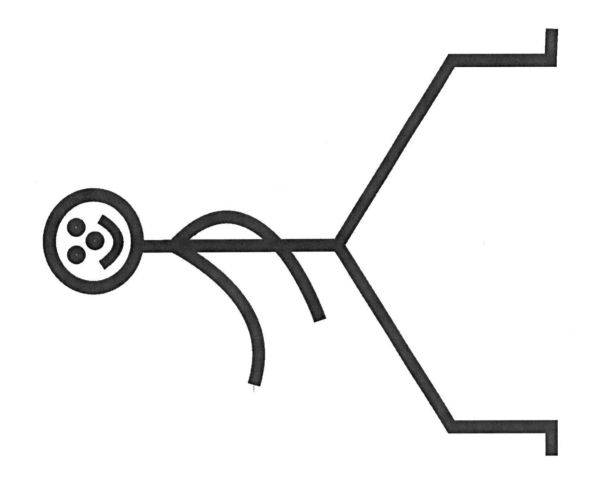

gorilla

April Merrilee

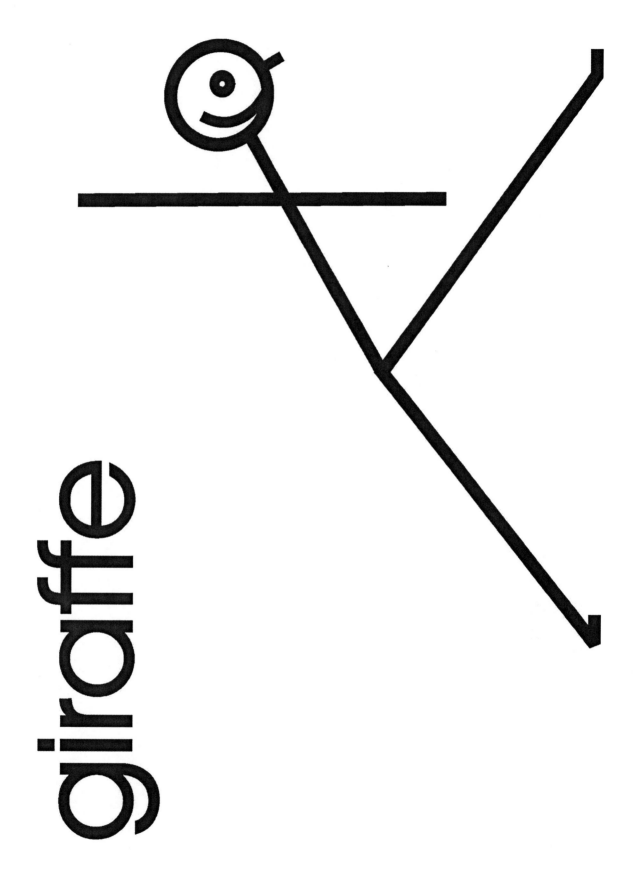

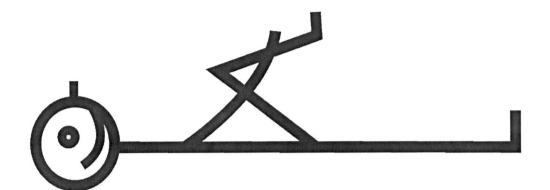

flamingo

April Merrilee

ostrich

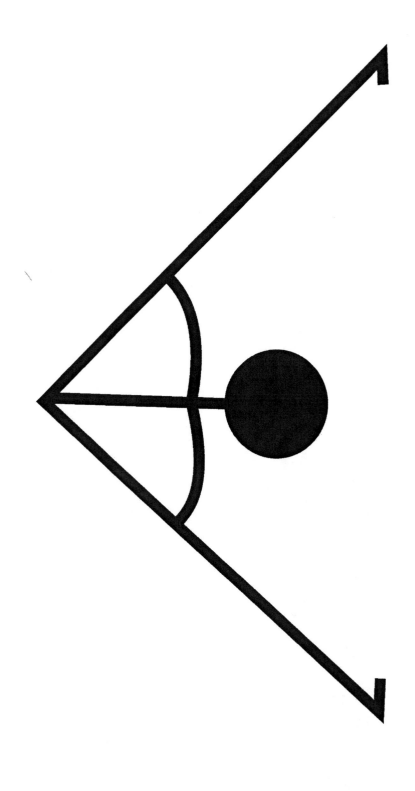

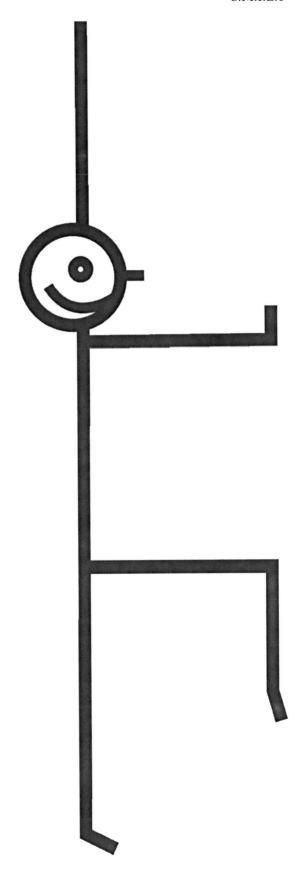

tiger

April Merrilee

monkey

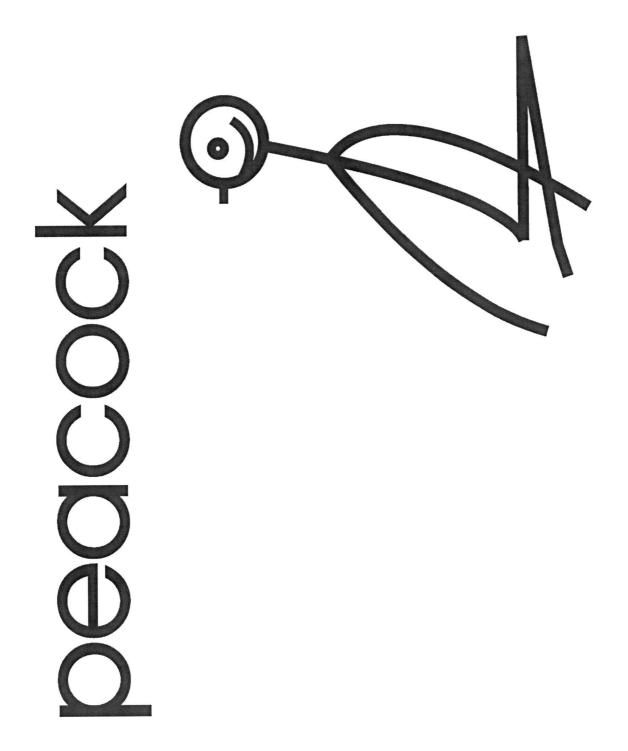

peacock

April Merrilee

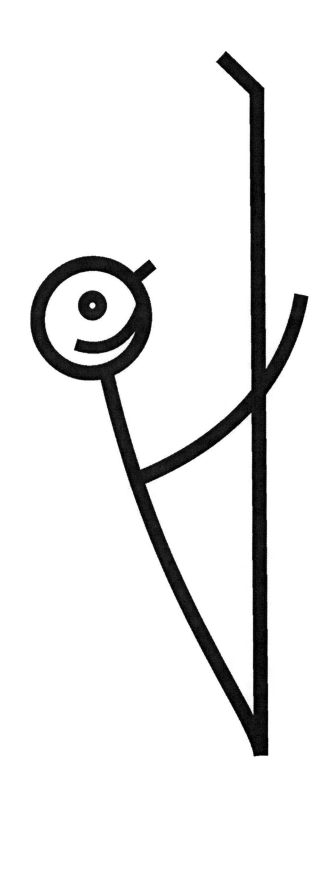

gator

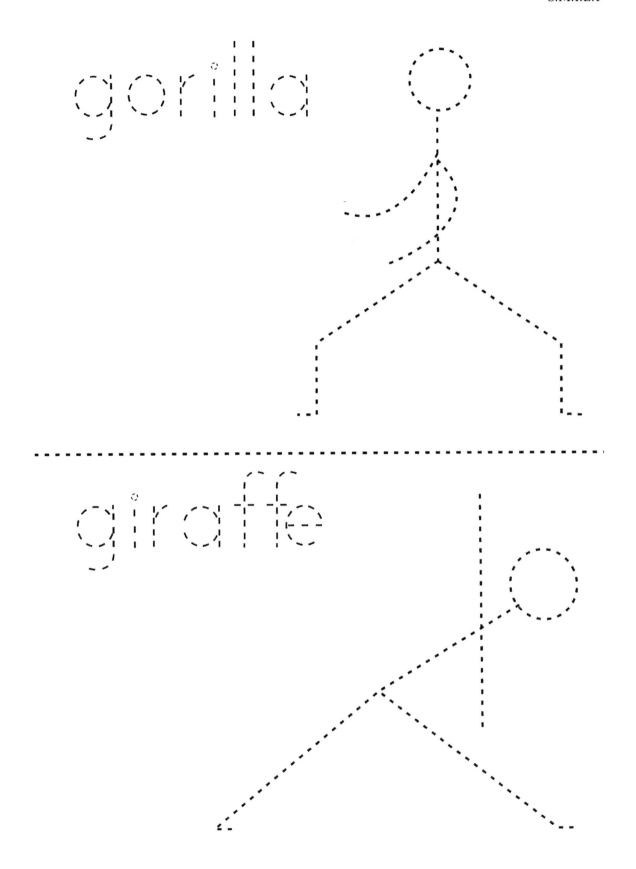

April Merrilee

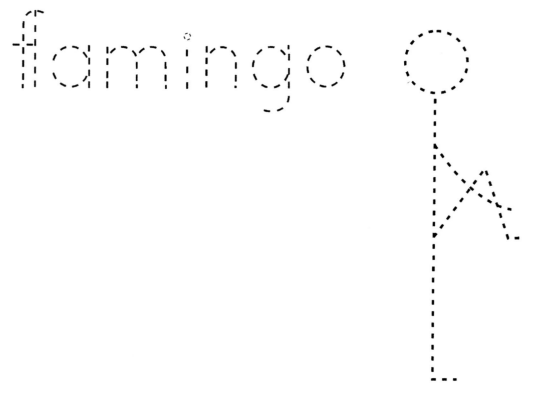

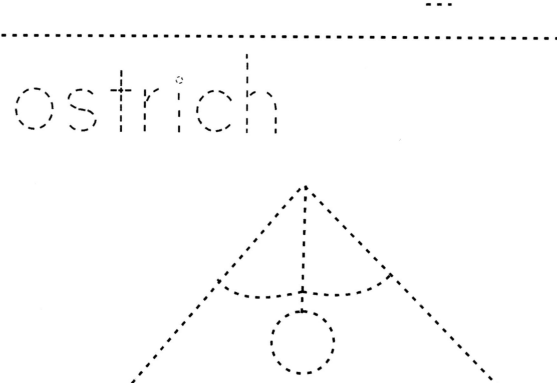

tiger

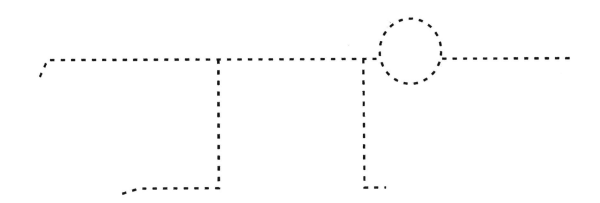

monkey

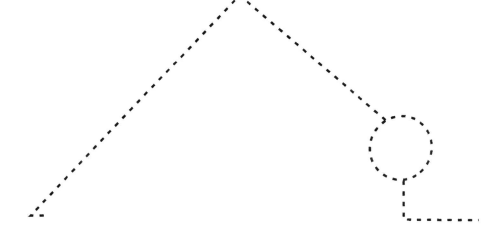

April Merrilee

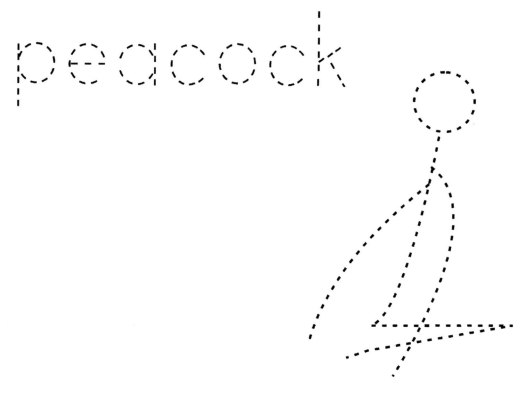

peacock

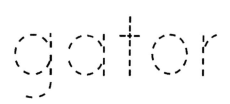

gator

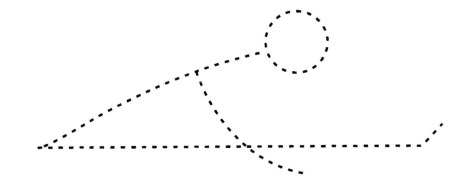

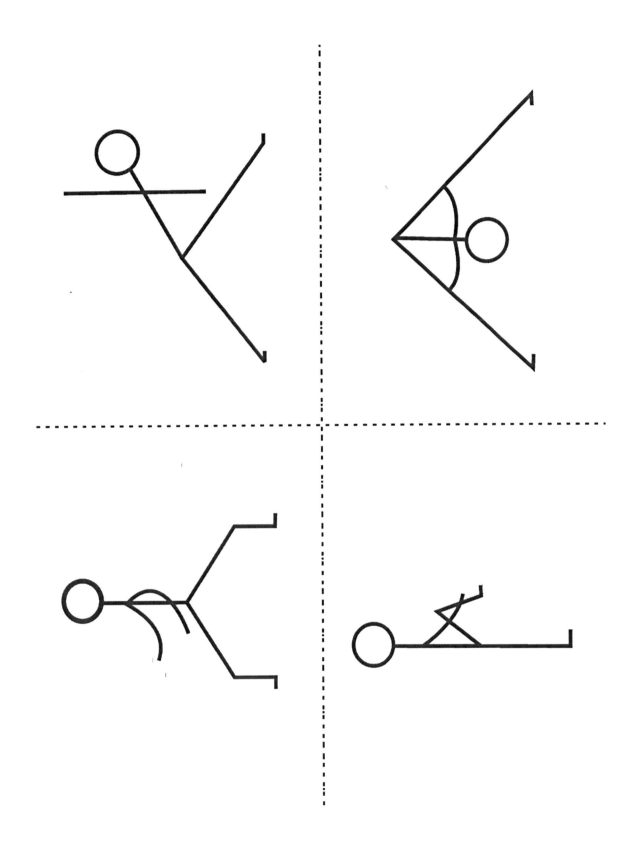

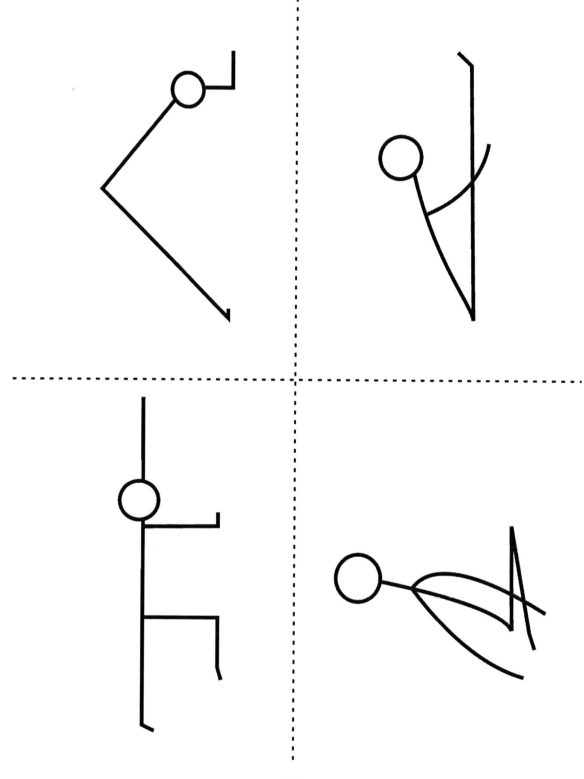

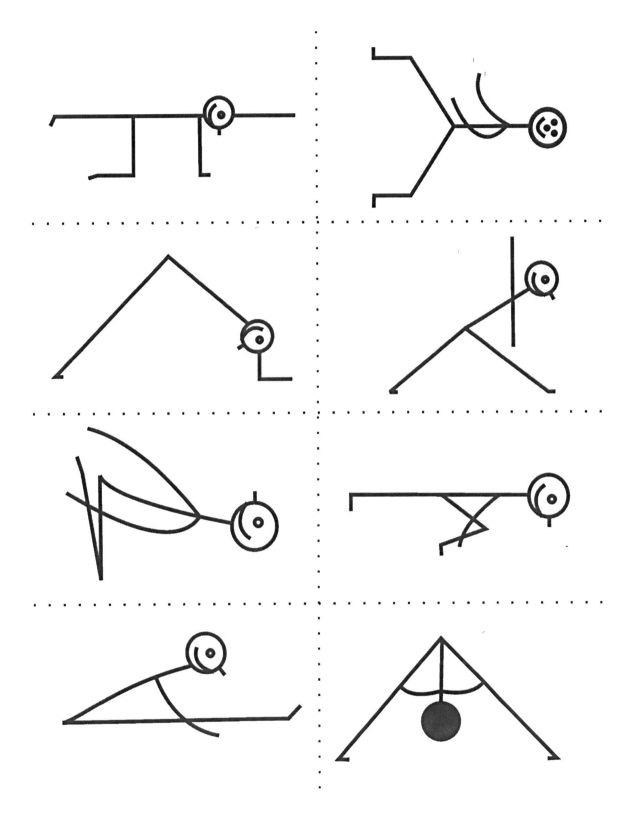

April Merrilee

tiger	gorilla
monkey	giraffe
peacock	flamingo
gator	ostrich

Basic Sentence Worksheet**Going On Safari**

Copy these sentences next to the correct drawing on the following page.

The gorilla is big.

The giraffe is tall.

A flamingo is pink.

The ostrich is a bird.

A tiger has stripes.

See the monkey swing.

The peacock is pretty.

The gator is green.

Challenge Sentence Worksheet: Match and copy next to the correct drawing!

I love to swing in the trees.

I like to eat nuts with my big hands.

I like to sleep in the winter.

I eat leaves from the tree tops.

I can stand on one leg.

I hunt for food in the jungle.

Watch me spread my beautiful feathers.

I get scared and try to hide.

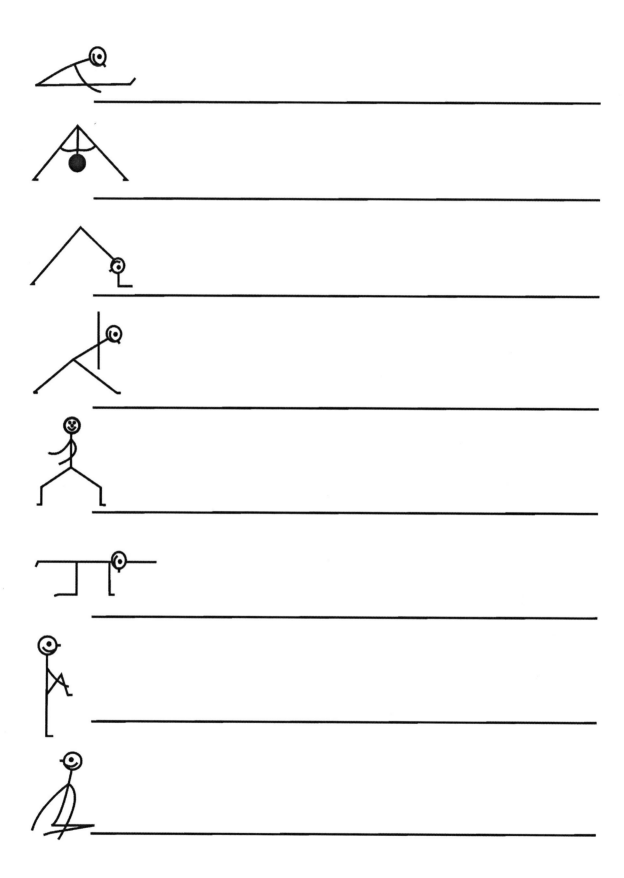

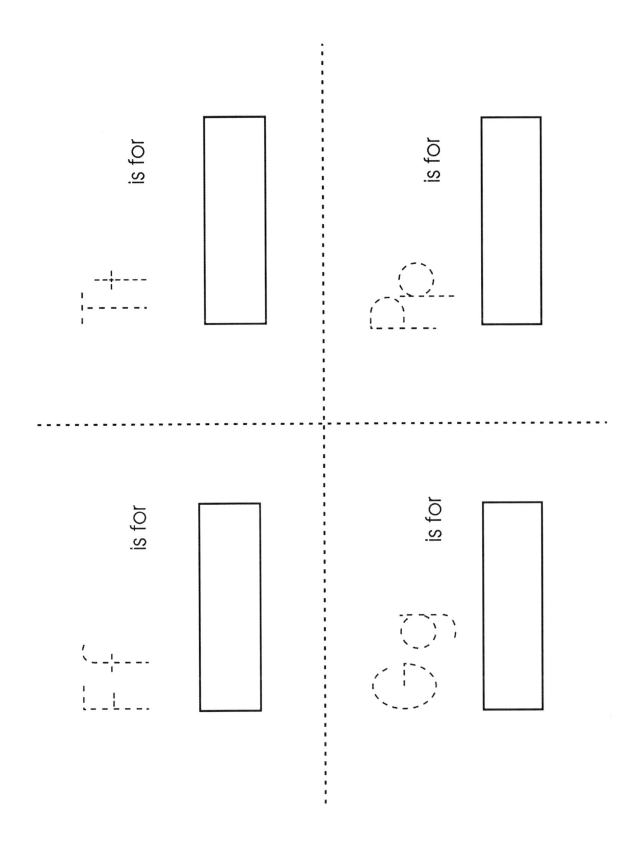

April Merrilee

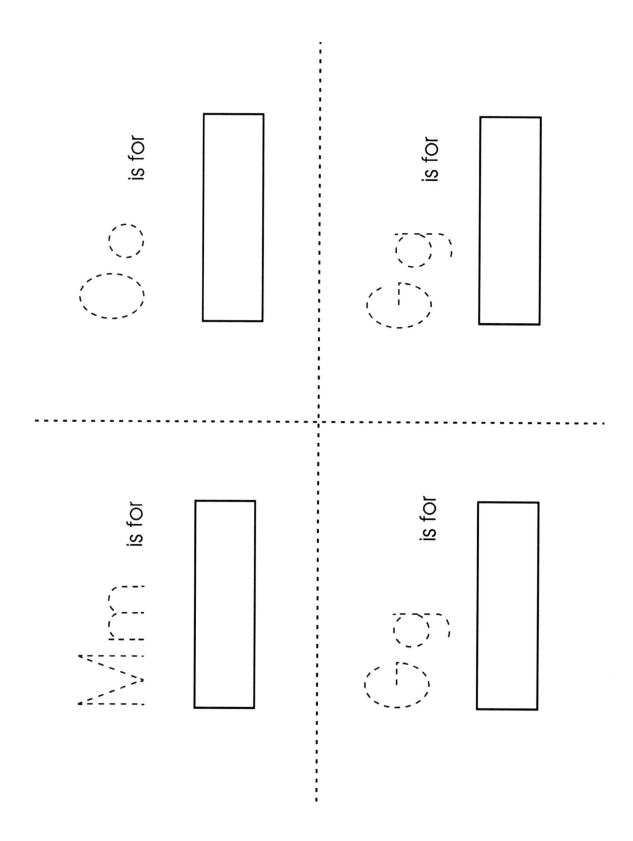

ROUTINE # 6: THE BUTTERFLIES

Lucy and Larry loved to catch butterflies. They would run around in their yard swinging their butterfly nets saying, "I caught a pink one!" and "I caught a purple one!" Show me how you swing your butterfly net **(imitation)**. What color is your butterfly? **(Kids take turns saying, "I caught a ...." Could include sign language for colors.)**

Lucy and Larry liked to keep their butterflies inside a glass jar. **(Mimic following motions:)** Let's get our jars out...and take off the lid. So, how many butterflies did we catch today? **(Pick a small number)** Teach sign language for "in". Okay, let's put them in the jar. **(Do sign for "in" for each butterfly while counting up to your chosen number.)**

All right now let's put the lid back on **(mimic motion)**. Good! That's how Lucy and Larry put their butterflies in, too. Just as they finished putting the lid on, their mother called them in for lunch. **(Mimic mother calling by cupping hands around mouth: "Lucy! Larry! Time for lunch!")**

So they ran into the house. **(Mimic running motion with arms.)** They ate a very good lunch **(teach sign for "eat")**. After lunch they were tired so they took nap. **(Mimic motion of hands to side of face for sleeping)**. But they forgot all about the poor butterflies, outside in their jar. The butterflies were flapping their wings against the glass saying, "Help! Help! We're stuck!" Pretty soon some of the animals in the neighborhood heard about the butterflies stuck in the jar, and everybody came over to try to get the jar open. Each animal tried using a different body part to get the jar open. Here's a song about all those animals trying to help.

Optional: Introduce each animal and have children guess which animal part they used. Can also teach sign language for the animal names.

LANGUAGE HIGHLIGHTS

- Sign language (colors, in, eat, sleep, animals)
- Gender pronouns (Mr./he ; Mrs./she)
- Future perfect verb tense
- Vocabulary: body parts
- /s/ blends
- /r/ sound
- final /g/

THE BUTTERFLIES
Sung to the tune of "Oh Susanna"

First verse:

Mr. Spider said, I will help you out
I will use my **legs** to open the jar
And set you free, no doubt!

Mr. Frog said, I will help you out
I will use my **mouth** to open the jar
And set you free, no doubt!

Mr. Ladybug said, I will help you out
I will use my **wings** to open the jar
And set you free, no doubt!

Mr. Crab said, I will help you out
I will use my **claws** to open the jar
And set you free, no doubt!

Mr. Lizard said, I will help you out
I will use my **tail** to open the jar
And set you free, no doubt!

Mr. Beaver said, I will help you out
I will use my **teeth** to open the jar
And set you free, no doubt!

Mr. Swan said, I will help you out
I will use my **beak** to open the jar
And set you free, no doubt!

Mr. Rabbit said, I will help you out
I will use my **ears** to open the jar
And set you free, no doubt.

(Tell children: But nobody could get the jar open. Mr. Rabbit said, we will call the ladies, maybe one of them can get it open.)

Second verse:

Mrs. Spider, she tried and tried and tried
She used her **legs** as best she could
But the butterflies stayed inside

Mrs. Frog, she tried and tried and tried
She used her **mouth** as best she could
But the butterflies stayed inside

Mrs. Ladybug, she tried..........
She used her **wings** as best she could....
(same as above)

Mrs. Crab, she tried..............
She used her **claws** as best she could....

Mrs. Lizard, she tried.........
She used her tail as best she could....

Mrs. Beaver, she tried.....
She used her teeth as best she could.....

Mrs. Swan, she tried.....
She used her **beak** as best she could...

Mrs. Rabbit, she tried and tried and tried
She used her **ears** as best she could
And opened that jar SO WIDE !!

Oh, those butterlies
They flew and flew and flew
They flapped their wings
And waved good-bye
Saying, "Many thanks to YOU!!"

Conclusion: while singing, do sign language for "thank you" and kids point to someone as fun surprise ending. Ask if the butterflies got out of the jar.

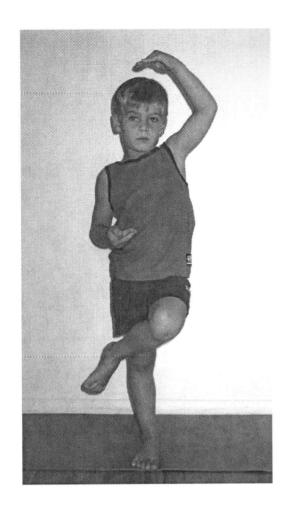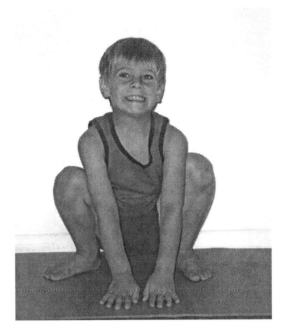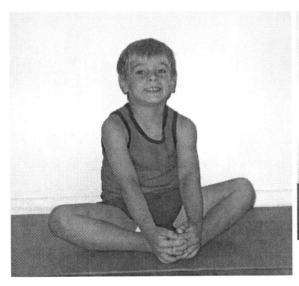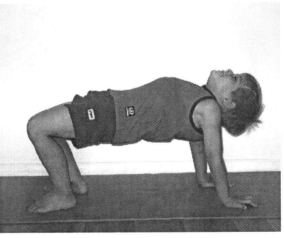

April Merrilee

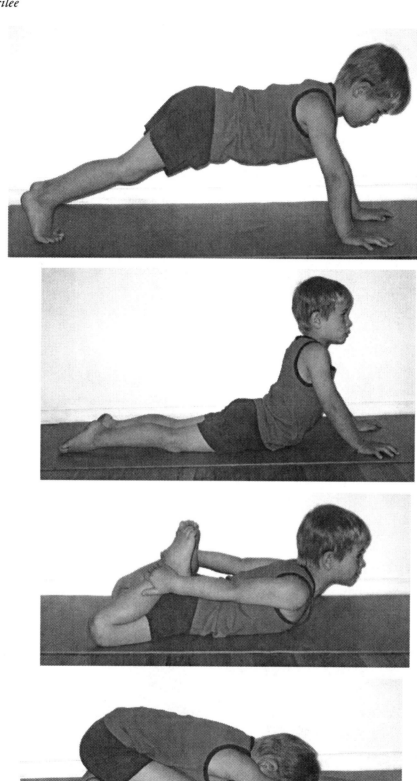

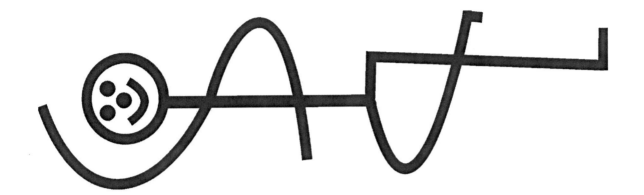

spider

April Merrilee

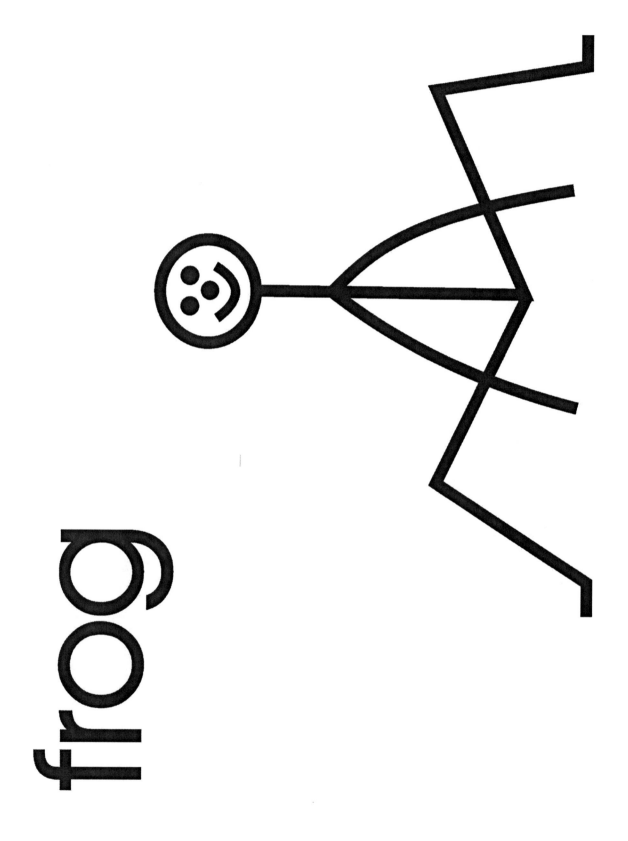

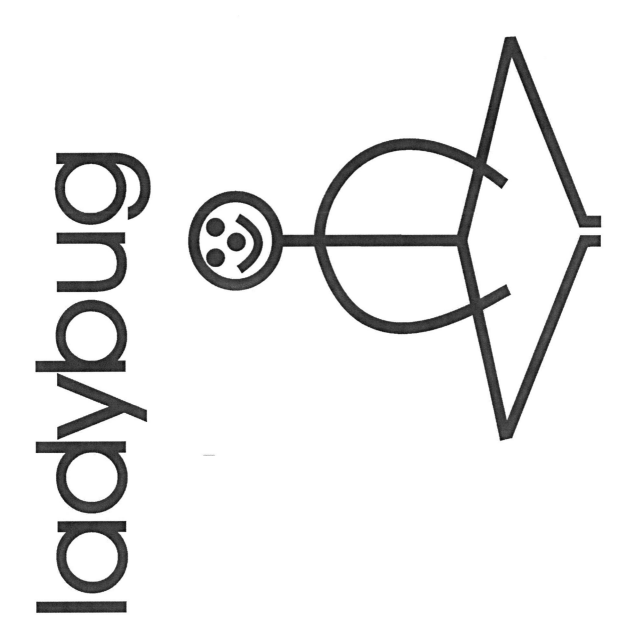

April Merrilee

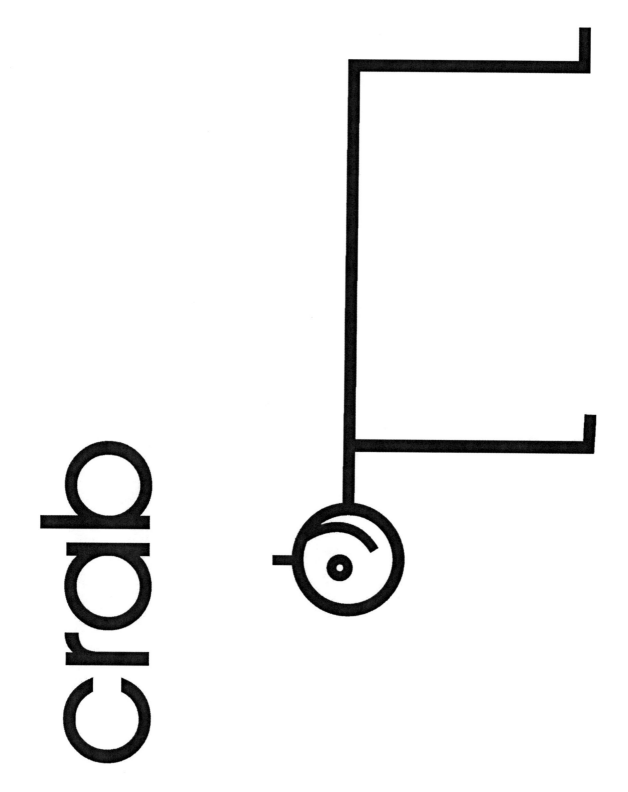

S.M.I.L.Y

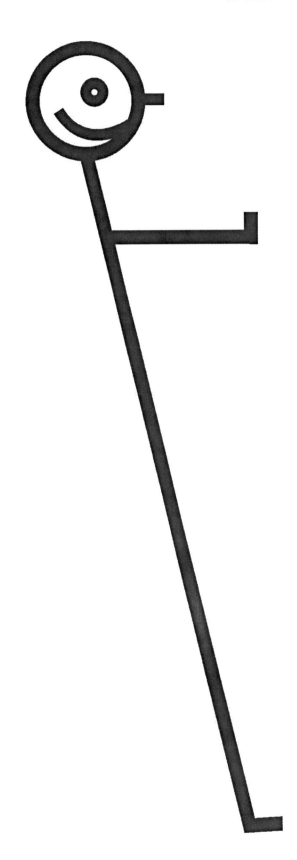

lizard

April Merrilee

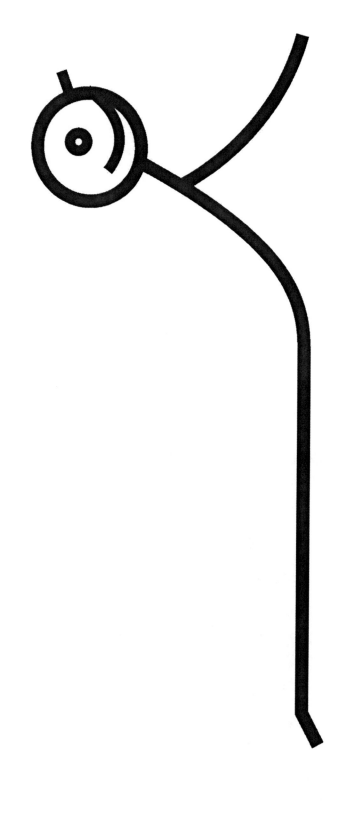

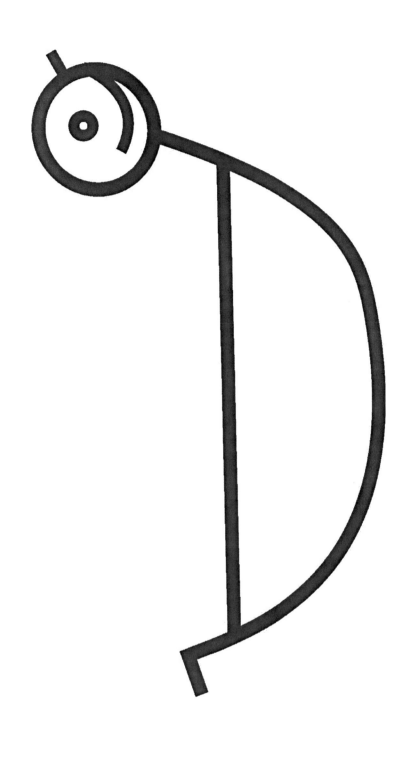

swan

April Merrilee

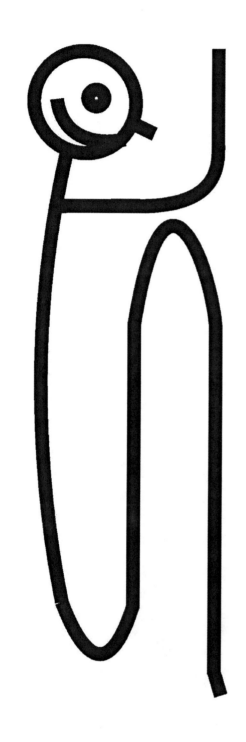

rabbit

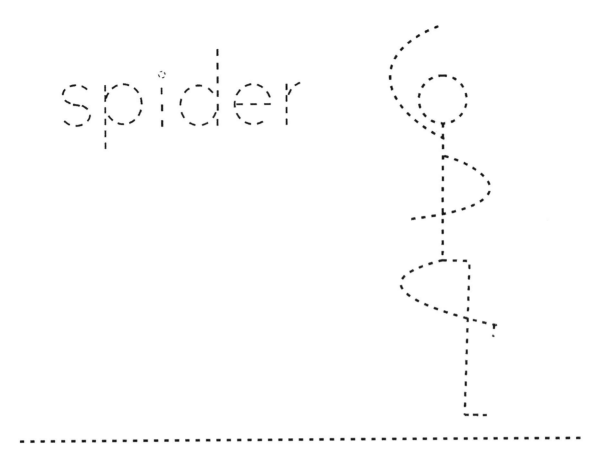
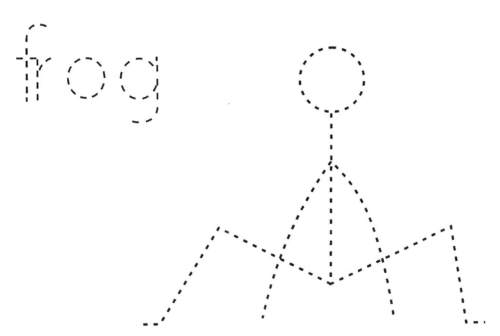

April Merrilee

ladybug

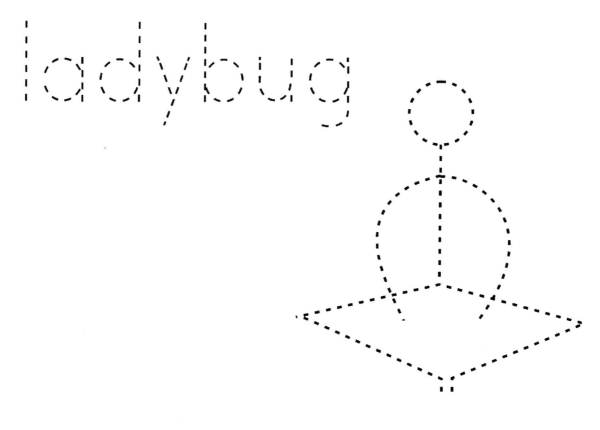

crab

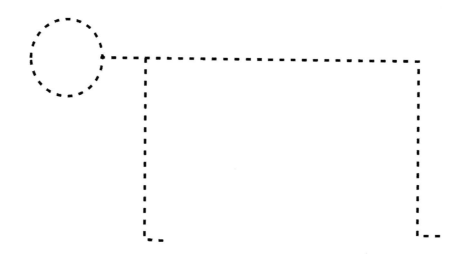

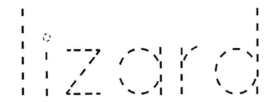

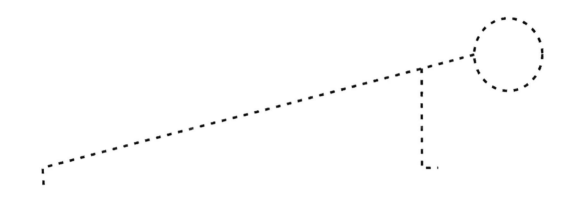

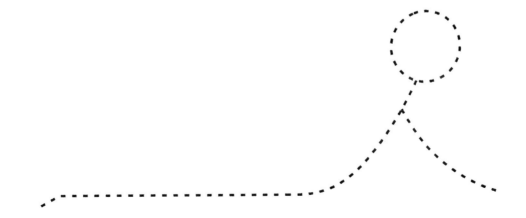

April Merrilee

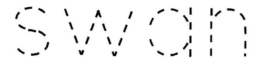

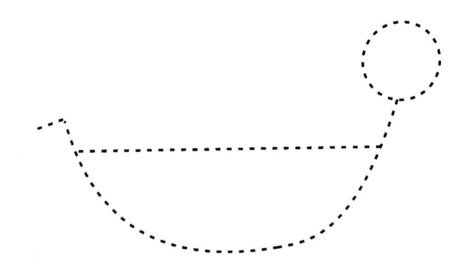

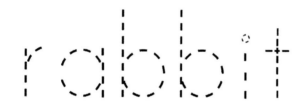

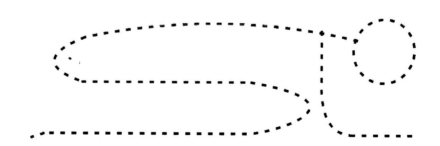

S.M.I.L.Y

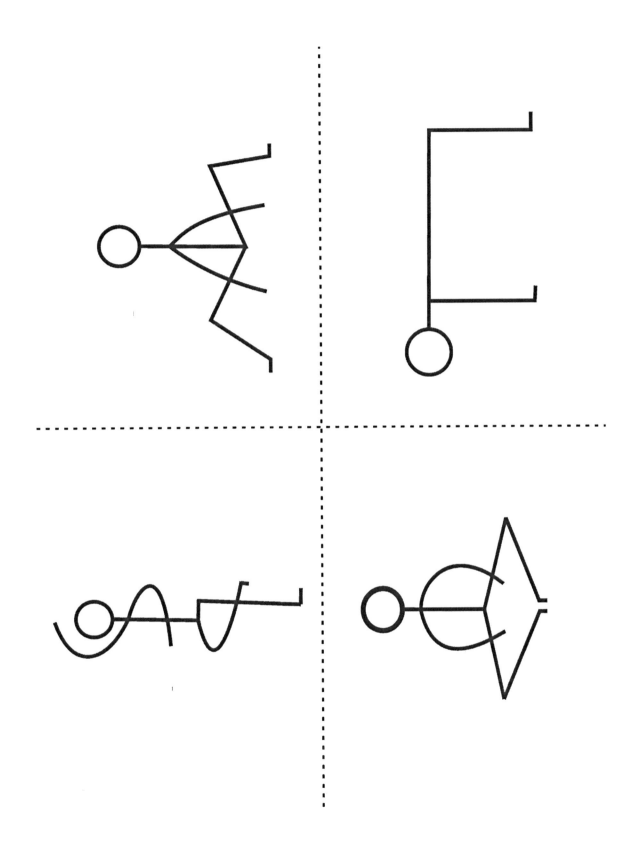

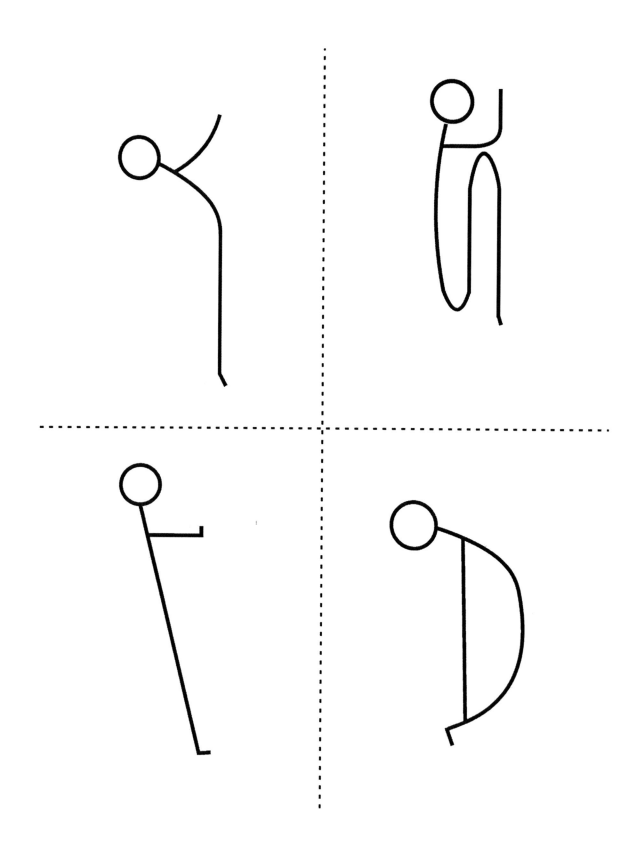

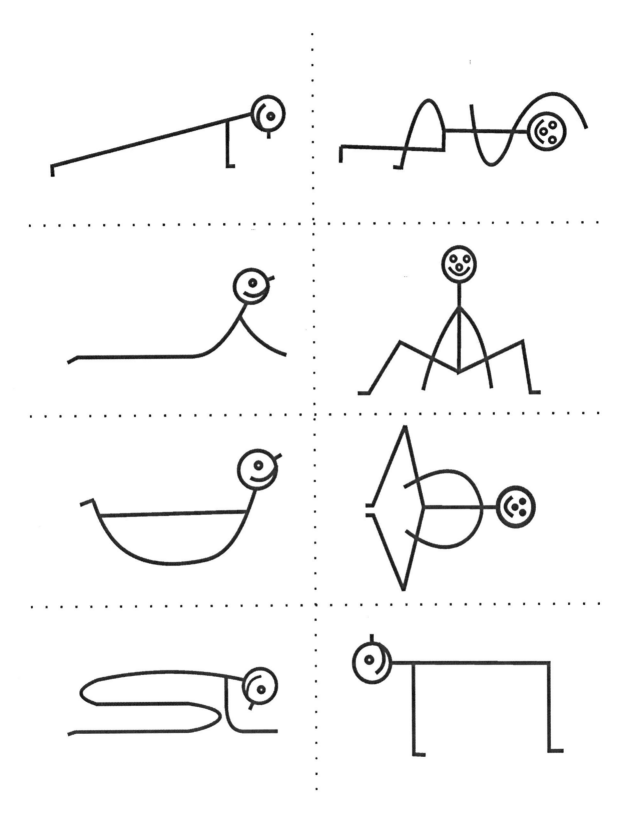

lizard	spider
beaver	frog
swan	ladybug
rabbit	crab

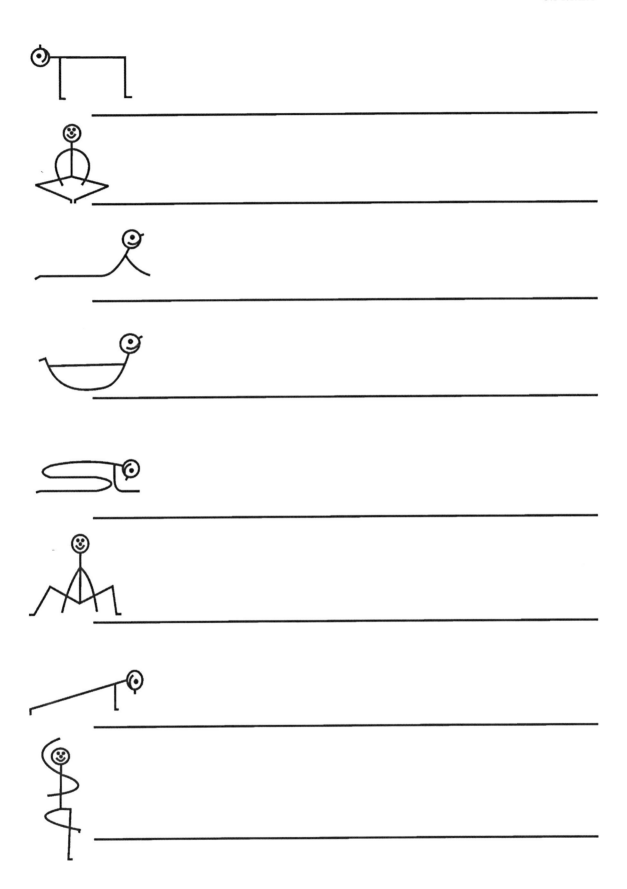

Basic Sentence Worksheet   The Butterflies

Copy these sentences next to the correct drawing on the following page.

The spider is black.

The frog is green.

A ladybug is red.

A crab has claws.

The lizard is long.

The beaver has big teeth.

The swan is white.

A rabbit is small.

Challenge Sentence Worksheet: Match and copy next to the correct drawing!

Look at my great big teeth!

I have eight legs - count them!

My tail is long and strong.

I can float on the water.

I have very small spots and wings.

I live on the sandy beach.

I like to sit on lily pads.

My ears are long and soft.

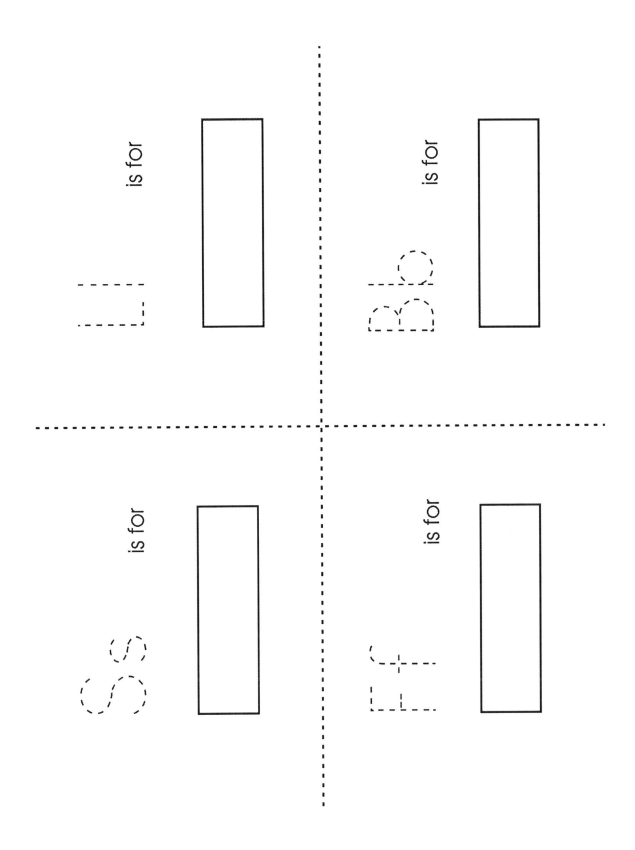

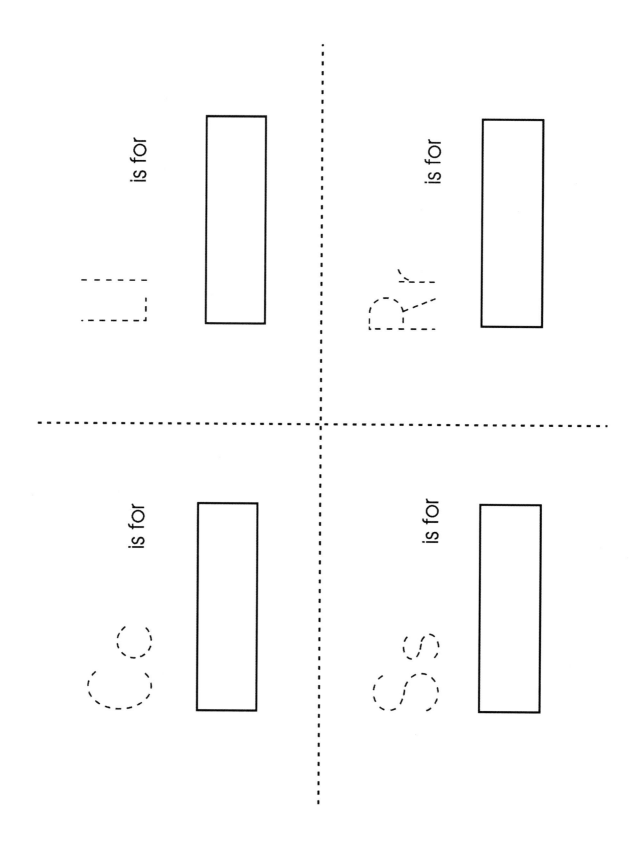

ROUTINE # 7: SWIMMING LESSONS

Once upon a time, in a kingdom far, far away, lived a lonely young frog. He knew he could become a fine prince some day, when the perfect fair maiden would
give him a kiss. But, alas, he could never meet any maidens because he was stuck in the castle with the king. You see, this castle was on an island in the middle of a big lake. Because he had spent all his time sitting with the king, this poor young frog had never learned to swim! One day the king told him it was time for young from to venture out in the world, fine a fair maiden, and become the fine prince he was meant to be. The frog was too embarrassed to tell the king that he did not know how to swim. After all, what kind of frog can't even swim across his own lake? I mean, REALLY!! So he sat by the lakeshore, trying to figure out how to swim. But every time he waded in, he just started to sink. The frog noticed there were lots of animals living at the lake, and they could all swim in one way or another. Each had its own special way of moving in the water that worked just right for them. For many days, he sat and watched these animals swim all around in the water. He saw the seagull bob; and the crawdad crawl; and the fish swish; and the snail scoot; and the swan glide; and the duck dive; and the otter flip; and the turtle kick! How much fun they were all having! More and more, he wanted to learn how to swim in his own special way. So, he got up the courage to ask the animals for swimming lessons to help him learn how to move his body in the water.

Optional: After Dreamer, ask children which animal taught the frog how to swim (turtle) and how did that animal move its body (kick). Have discussion about all the ways the other animals move their body, and if kids could learn how to swim like any of those animals.

LANGUAGE HIGHLIGHTS FOR SWIMMING SONG

- Action words - new verbs (bob, crawl, swish, scoot, glide, drive, flip, kick, strive)
- Vocabulary: unfamiliar marine animals
- Rhyming words
- /s/ blends
- Initial /f/ sound
- Contractions

April Merrilee

SWIMMING LESSONS
Sung to the tune of "Camptown Races"

Intro: Sing while standing and clapping or crossing midline:

How I want to learn to swim
What should I say?
Maybe I can learn from them
Then I'll swim away

Repeat intro between verses

First verse - first melody line

Seagull can you teach me how
To bob with you
I'll go in the water now
Show me what to do

Second verse - next melody line:

I saw the **seagull bob**
Wish I could do the job
How can I begin to move like him
When will I learn how to swim

Crawdad can you teach me how
To crawl with you
I'll go in the water now
Show me what to do

I saw the **crawdad crawl**
He's having such a ball !
How can I begin to move like him
When will I learn how to swim

Fish can you teach me how
To swish with you
(repeat same lines, each animal)

I saw the **fish swish**
This is my only wish
(repeat same lines, each animal)

Snail can you teach me how
To scoot with you

I saw the **snail scoot**
It looks like such a hoot

Swan can you teach me how
To glide with you

I saw the **swan glide**
Right to the other side

Duck can you teach me how
To dive with

I saw the **duck dive**
That's how to be alive

Otter can you teach me how
To flip with you

I saw the **otter flip**
He can take any trip

Turtle can you teach me how
To kick with you

I saw the **turtle kick**
Think I can do the trick
Now I can begin to move like him
Watch me, I know how to swim

Conclusion: Ask children if the frog learned to swim. Which animal helped him finally learn how?

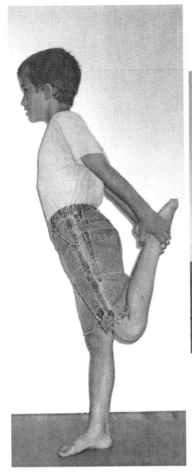
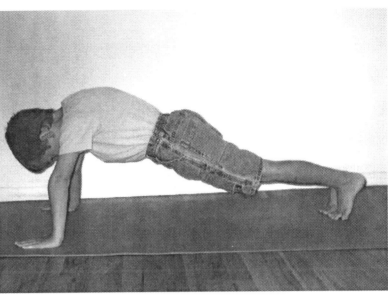
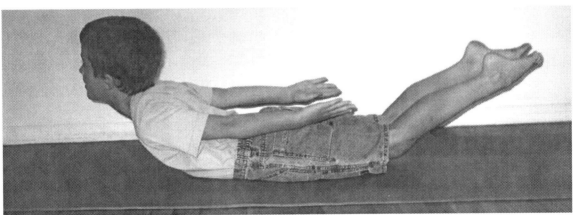
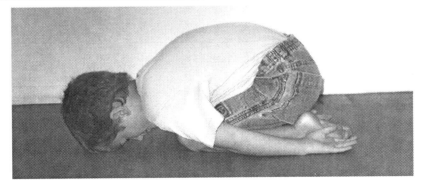

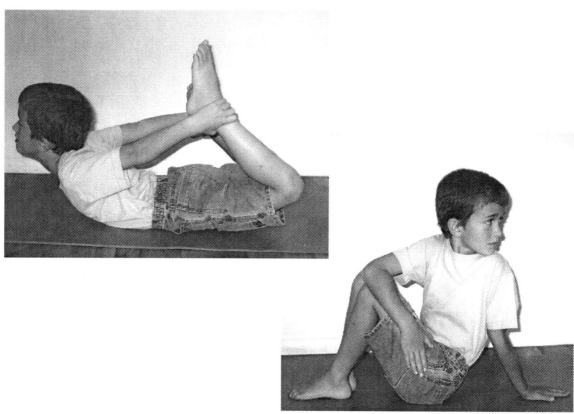
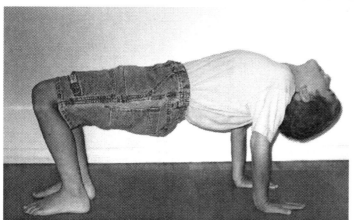
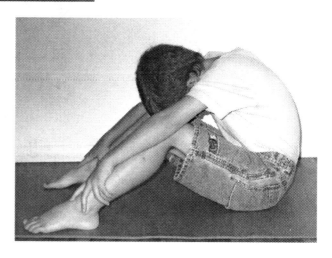

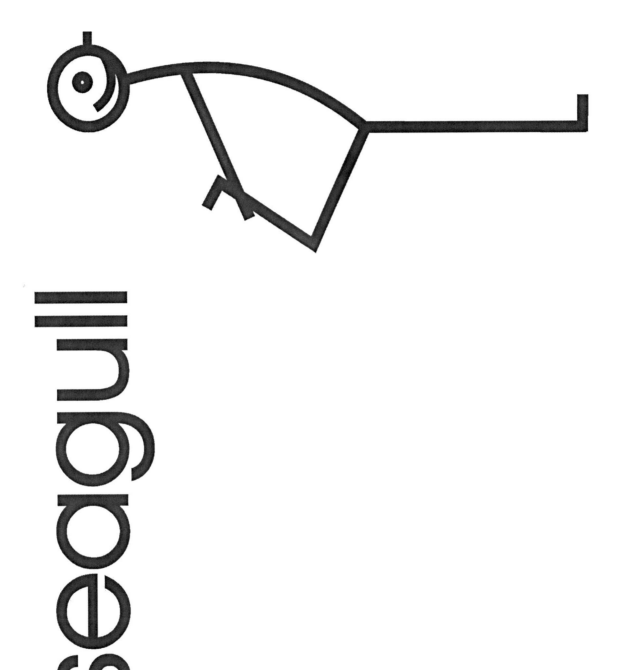

seagull

April Merrilee

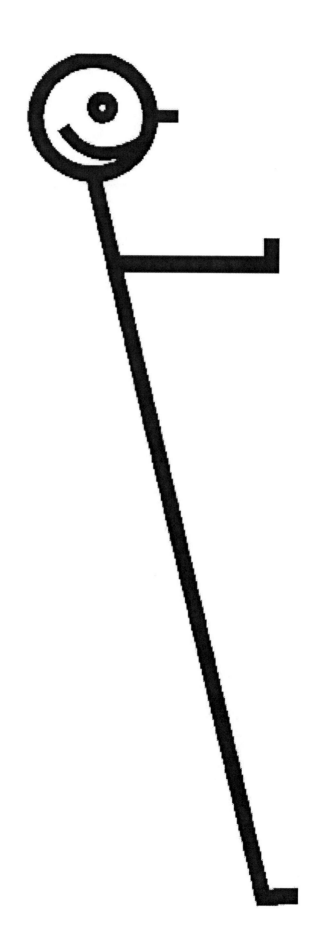

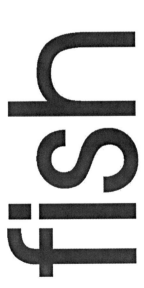
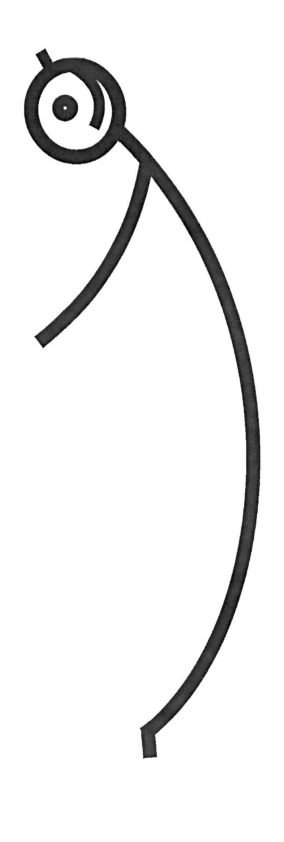

fish

April Merrilee

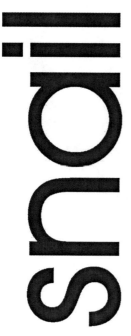
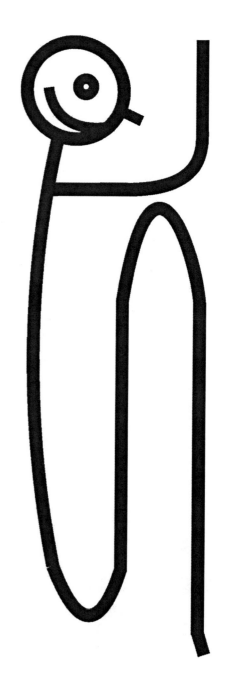

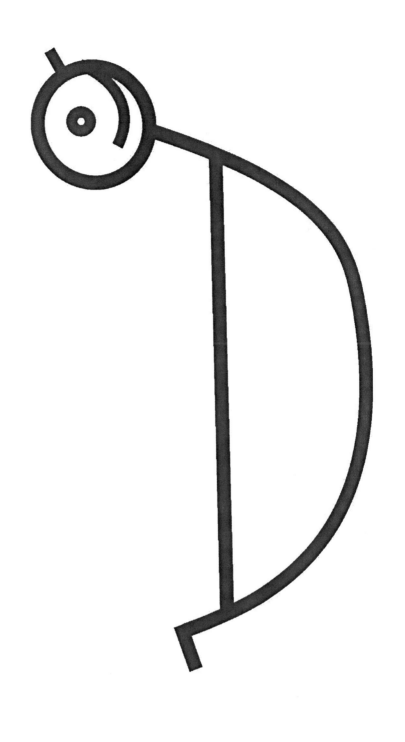

swan

April Merrilee

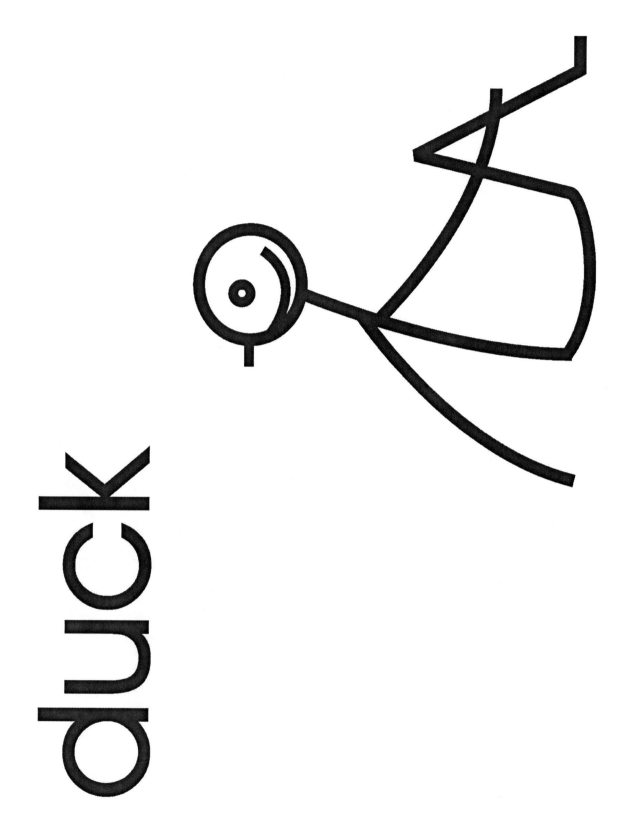

duck

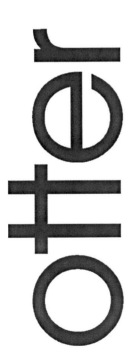
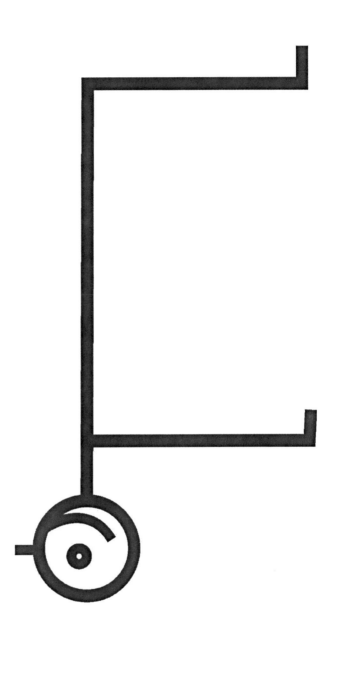

April Merrilee

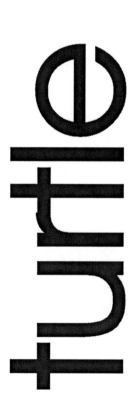
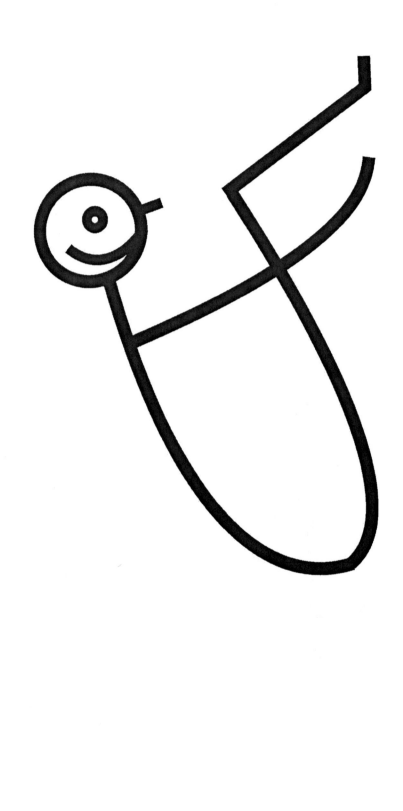

seagull

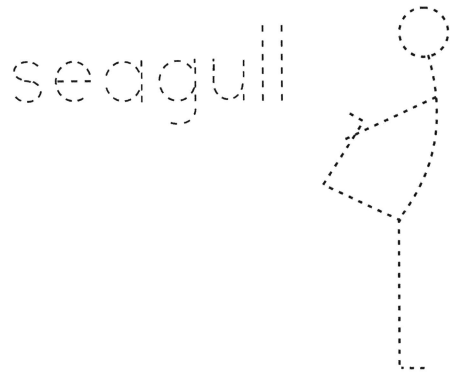

---

crawdad

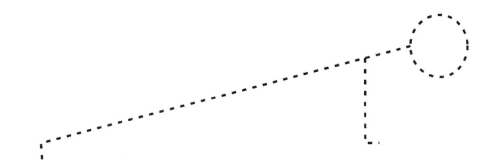

April Merrilee

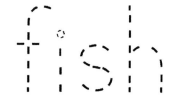

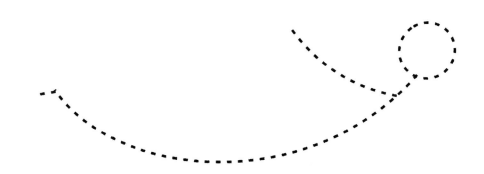

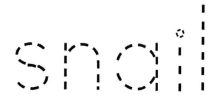

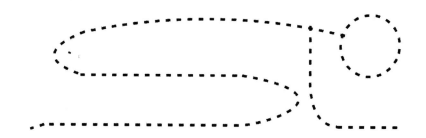

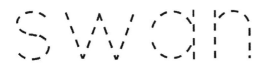

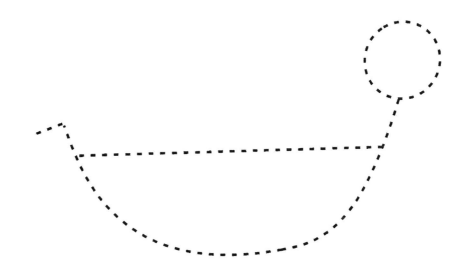

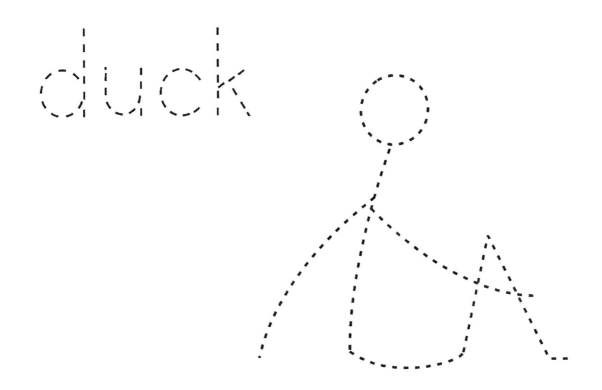

April Merrilee

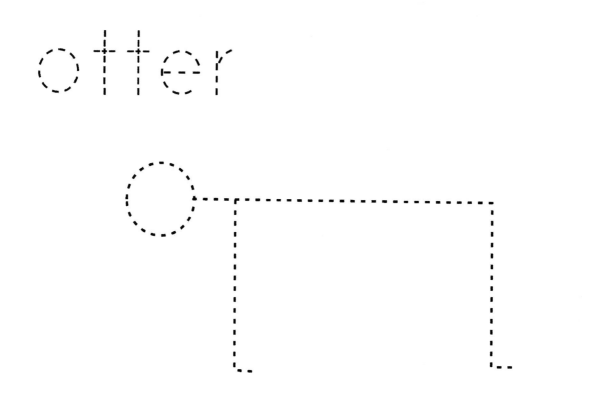

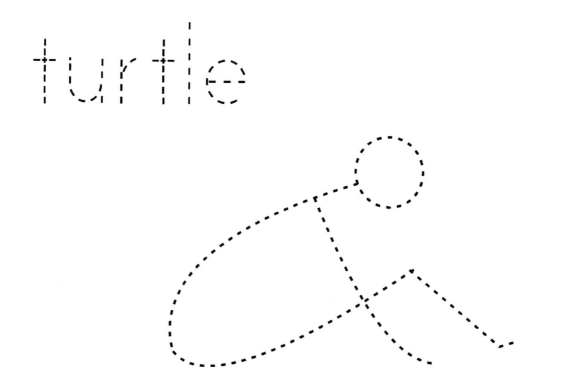

S.M.I.L.Y

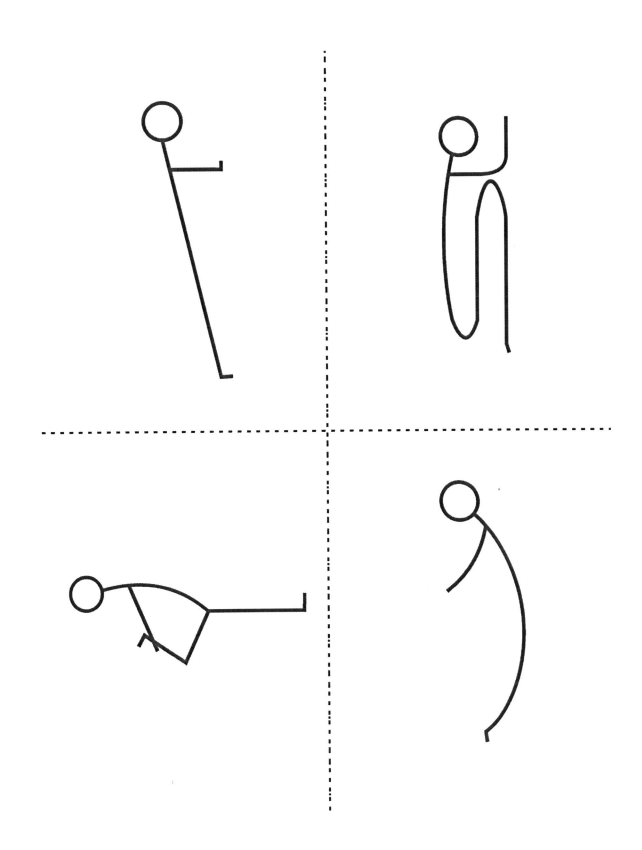

April Merrilee

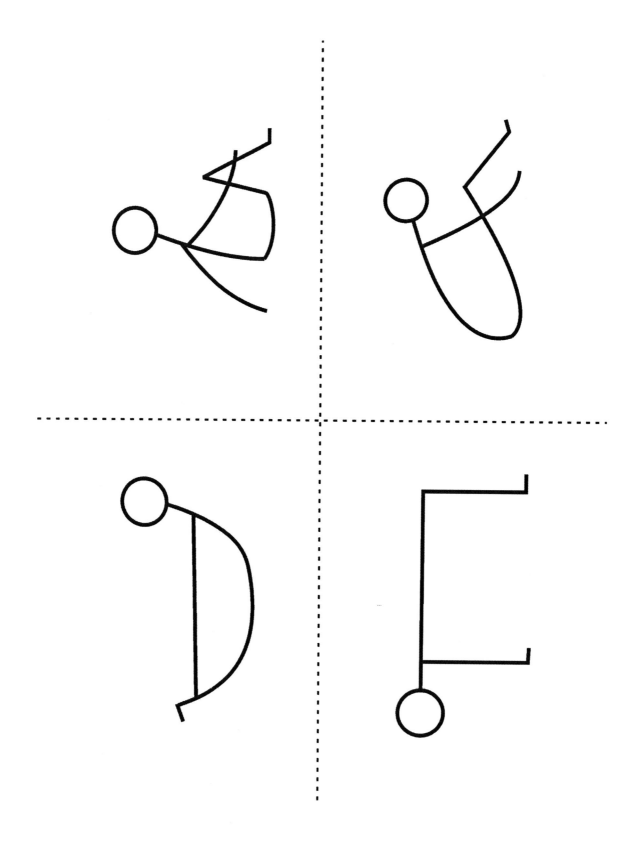

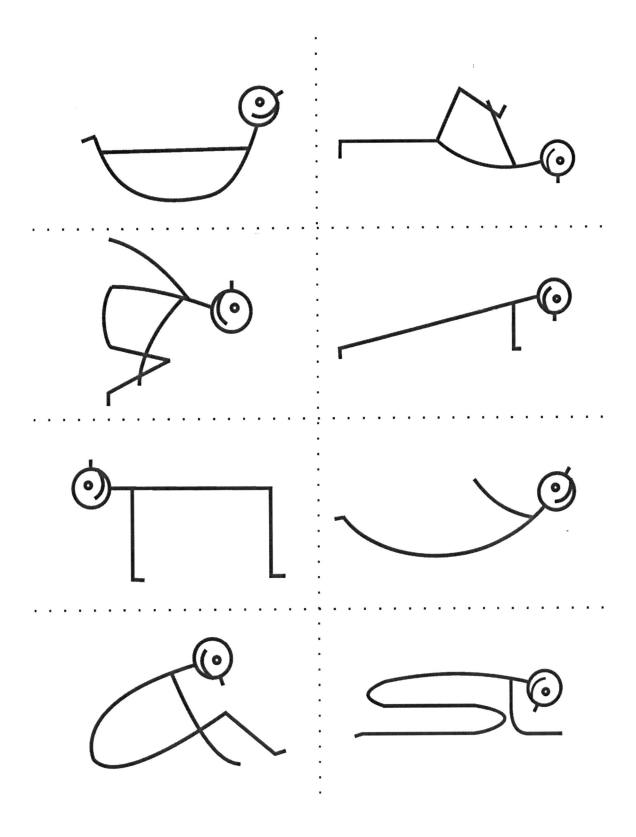

swan	seagull
duck	crawdad
otter	fish
turtle	snail

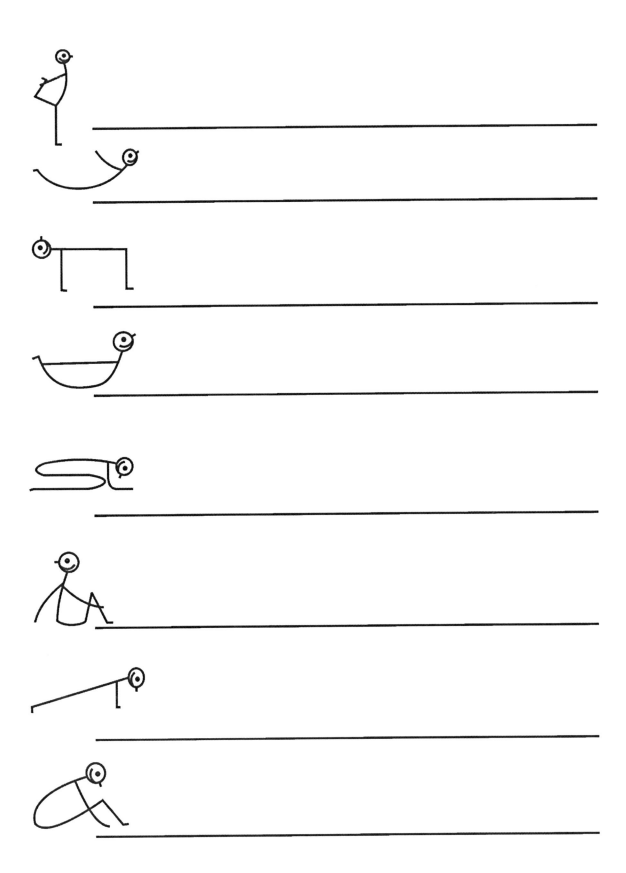

Basic Sentence Worksheet   Swimming Lessons

Copy these sentences next to the correct drawing on the following page.

A seagull is a bird.

A crawdad is red.

The fish has fins.

A snail is small.

The swan is pretty.

The duck is brown.

The otter is fun.

The turtle is slow.

Challenge Sentence Worksheet: Match and copy next to the correct drawing!

I have a long white neck.

My shell is large and very hard.

You can find me at the seashore.

My babies swim behind me.

I swim around all day long.

I crawl through the mud.

Watch me flip in the water.

I live inside a tiny shell.

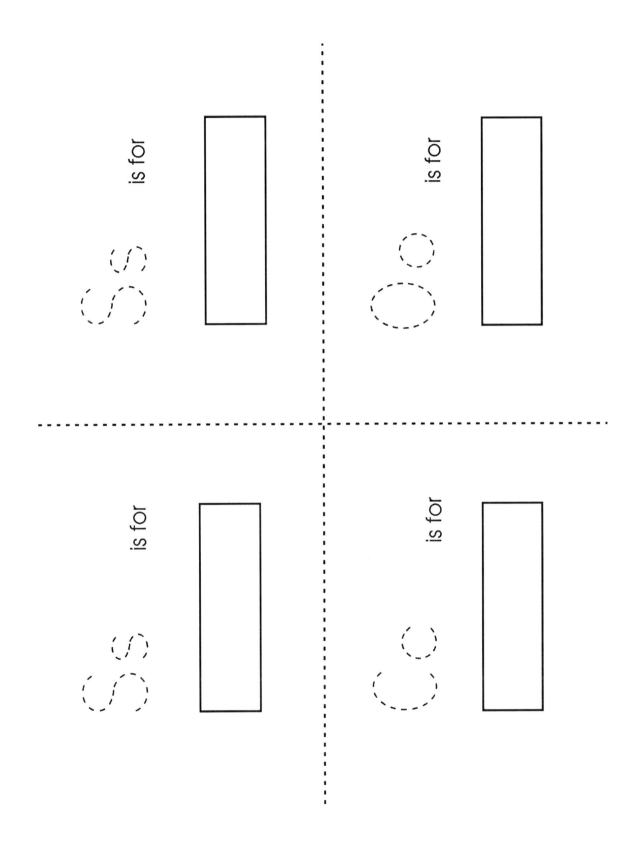

April Merrilee

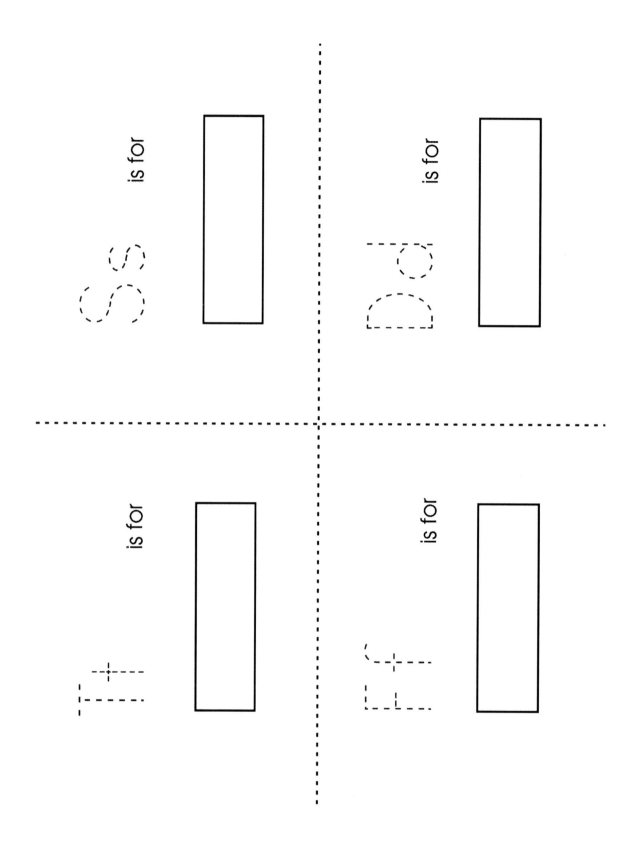

ROUTINE # 8 : MAMA DUCK

It was spring down on the farm. Do you know what happens in springtime? All the animals have their babies! Did you know that many animals have special names for their babies? What do we call a baby cat? What do we call a baby dog? That's right, the cats were having their kittens, and the dogs were having their puppies. What do we call a baby chicken? (chicks) How about a baby pig? Hint: Winnie the Pooh has a baby pig for a friend, who is that little pink guy? (piglet). The cows were having their calves. And what do we call a baby sheep (those cute little fuzzy animals)? That's right lambs. Now, these next two are pretty tricky! Does anybody know the name of a baby horse? A baby horse is called a foal. And here's one you may never have heard before: what do you call a baby swan? A baby swan has a very different name; it is called a cygnet. Can you say that word?

Okay, here's an easier one. What do you call a baby duck? That's right, a duckling. And ducklings come out of eggs, don't they? Well, this spring Mama Duck was hatching her eggs. How many eggs do you think she had in her nest? Wow, that's a lot of eggs! Can anybody tell me how those baby ducklings get out of their eggs? Yup, they have to crack that shell. And what body part do they use to break that shell open? Their beaks! Well, all of Mama Ducks' eggs hatched but one. While her babies were learning to swim and eat, she still had one last egg sitting in her nest, and it just wouldn't hatch! Well, pretty soon all the animals on the farm heard about this baby duckling that just wasn't breaking out of its shell. They thought and thought of a way to help Mama and her baby. Finally they decided that each animal would bring the baby a special present, so he would have to come out of its shell to see all their gifts. Each animal brought their very favorite thing over to the nest, and Mama Duck sang this song to her baby, trying to get him to come out and see all the wonderful presents their friends had brought.

Optional: Discuss as part of story what all the animals would bring as further introduction to song. For example, ask, "What would be the horse's favorite thing?"

or "What does the pig like to roll around in?", etc. Helpful for younger children to learn lyrics before singing.

Conclusion: After Dreamer, ask children which of the presents they think the baby duckling liked best / which one made him crack his shell and come out.

LANGUAGE HIGHLIGHTS

- Sign language for farm animals during story time
- Vocabulary: names of animal offspring
- Final /ing/ sound
- Final /t/ sound
- Final /g/ sound
- Association: matching animals with objects (presents)

MAMA DUCK
Sung to the tune of "Clementine" (Oh my darling...)

First verse:

Oh my duckling, oh my duckling
Oh my duckling, crack your shell
You might like what
Horse has brought you
Better look 'cause I won't tell.

Oh my duckling, oh my duckling
Oh my duckling, crack your shell
You might like what
Cow has brought you
Better look 'cause I won't tell

(repeat verse, inserting animals)

....you might like what
Cat has brought you......

....you might like what
Dog has brought you....

....you might like what
Swan has brought you...

....you might like what
Sheep has brought you

....you might like what
Pig has brought you

....you might like what
Frog has brought you

Second verse:

Oh my duckling, oh my duckling
Oh my duckling, take a peek
Your friend **horse** has
Hay to give you
It is time to use your beak.

Oh my duckling, oh my duckling
Oh my duckling, take a peek
Your friend **Cow** has
Milk to give you
It is time to use your beak.

(Insert animals and objects)

...Your friend **Cat** has
Toys to give you..........

...Your friend **Dog** has
Bones to give you...

...Your friend **Swan** has
Fish to give you...

...Your friend **Sheep** has
Wool to give you...

...Your friend **Pig** has
Mud to give you...

...Your friend **Frog** has
Bugs to give you...

Conclusion: Oh my duckling, oh my duckling,
Oh my duckling, he broke through
All the presents were so special
He just had to say, "Thank you"

Use sign for "thank you" and point to someone

April Merrilee

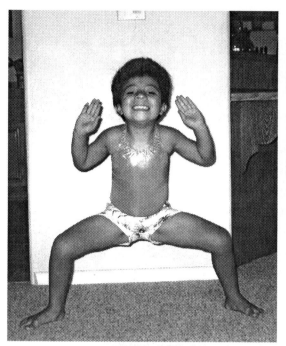
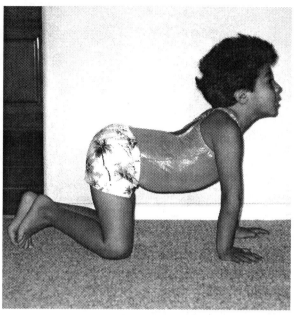
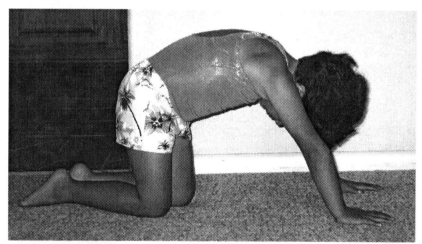
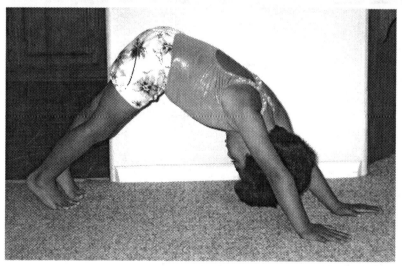

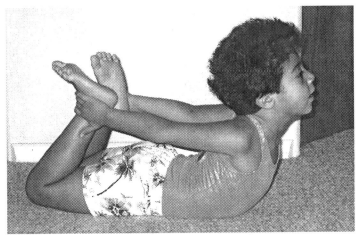
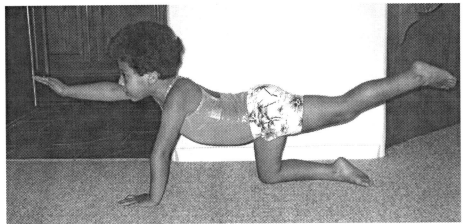
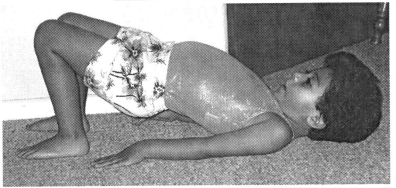
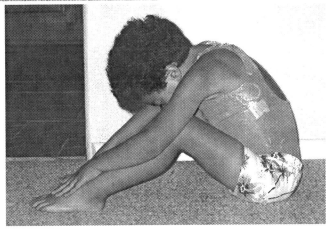

April Merrilee

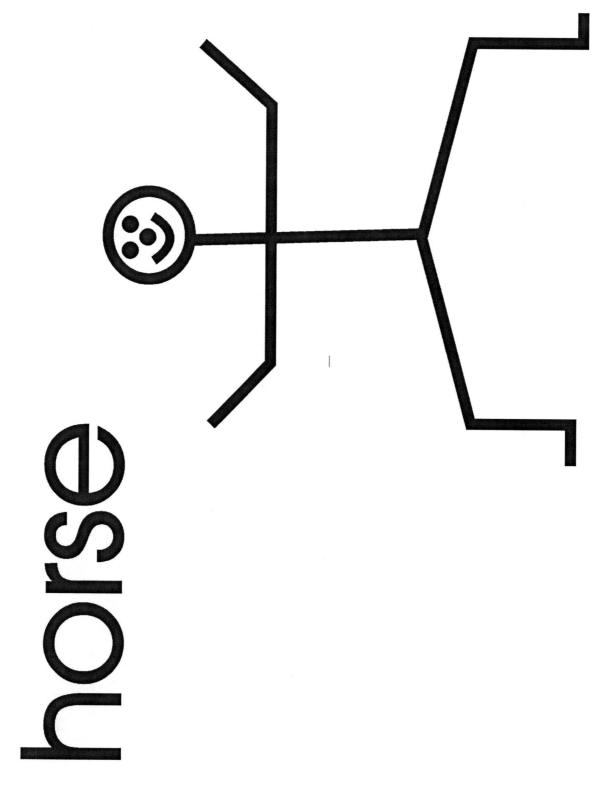

horse

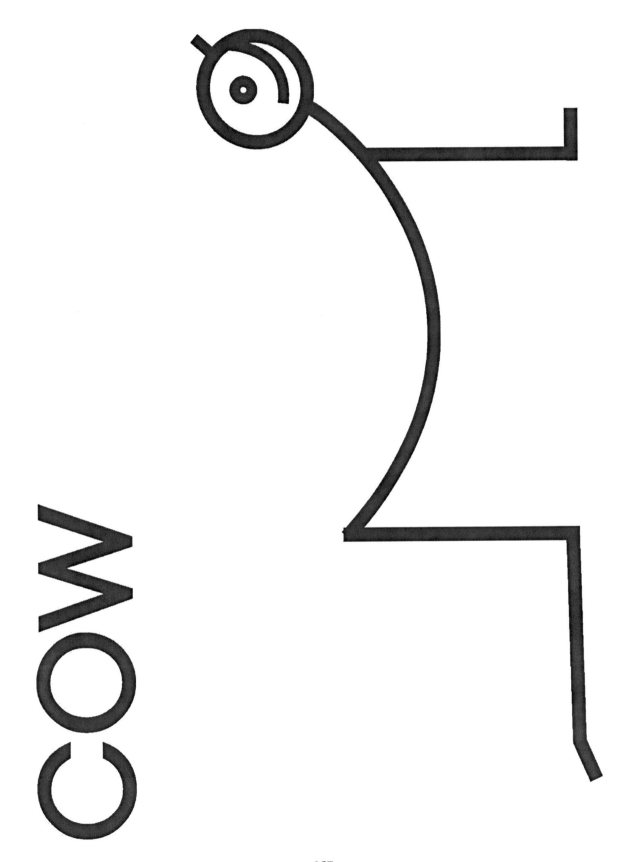

April Merrilee

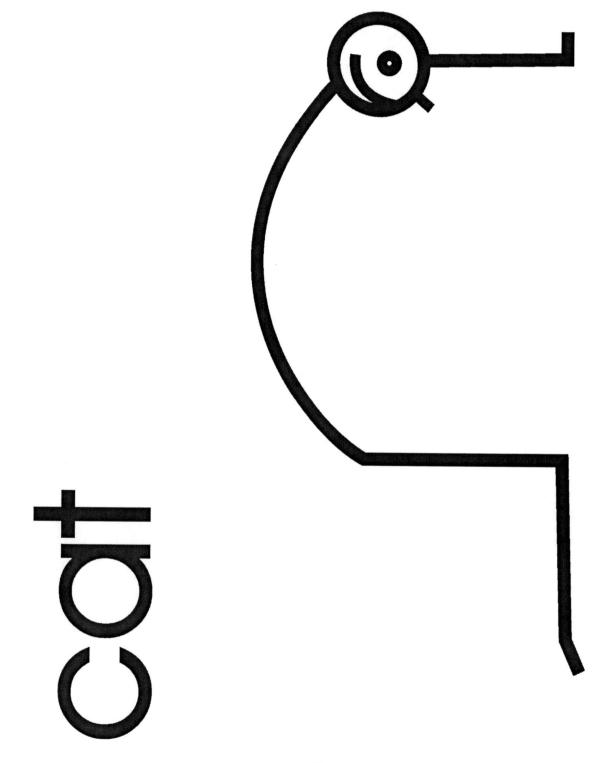

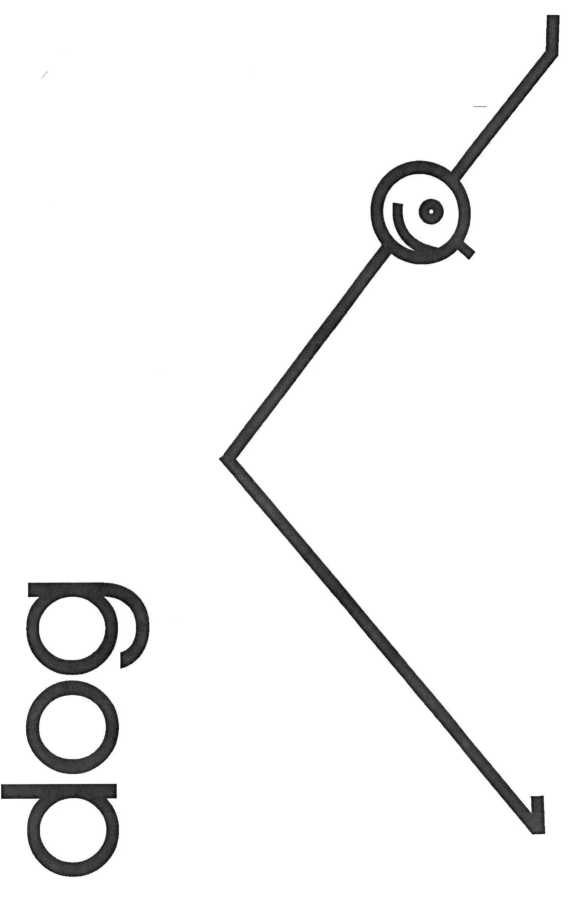

April Merrilee

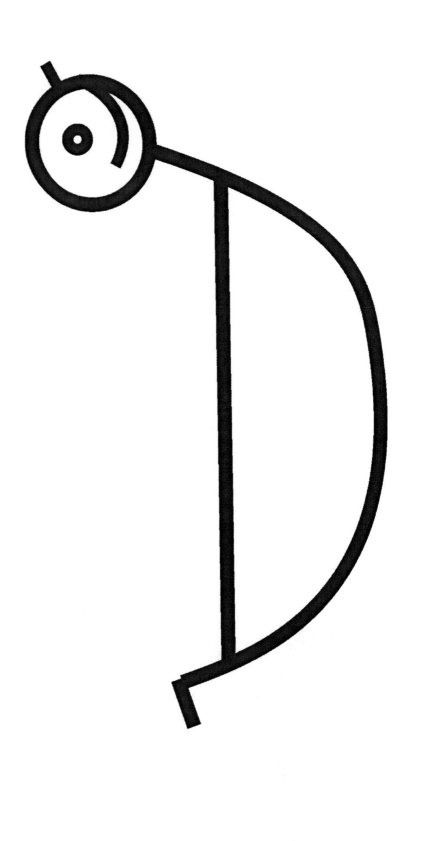

swan

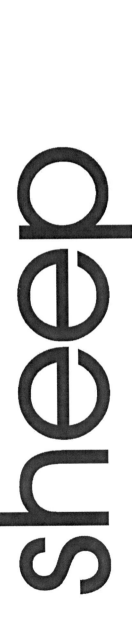
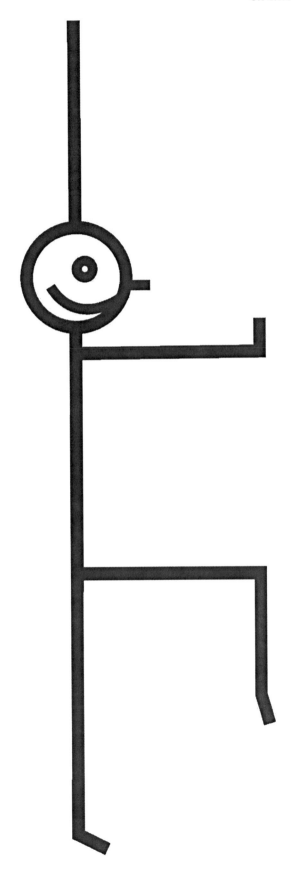

April Merrilee

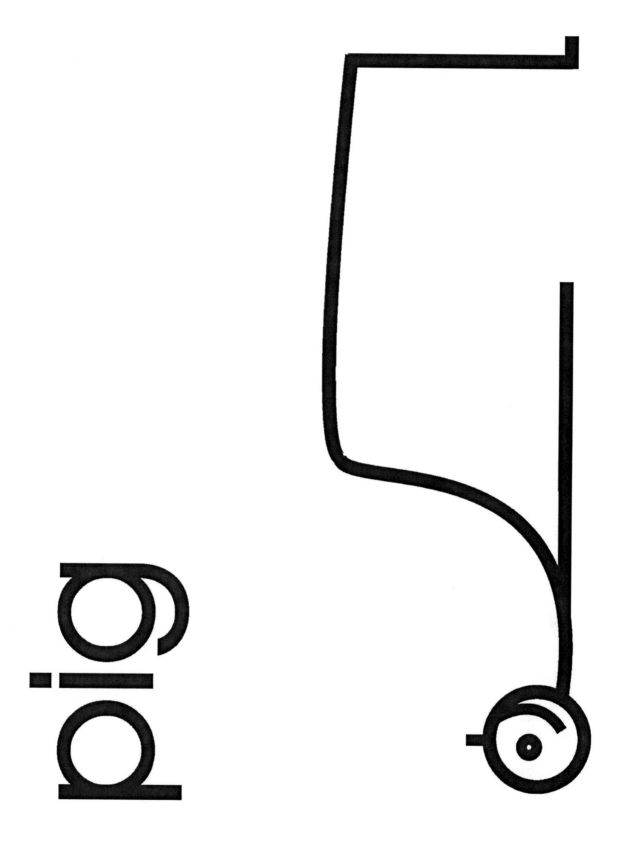

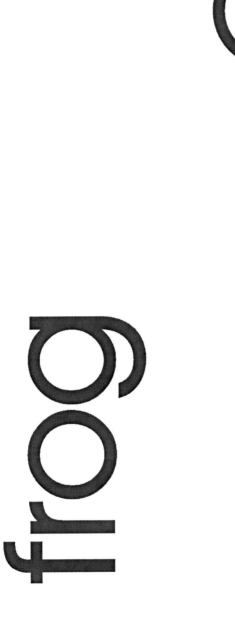
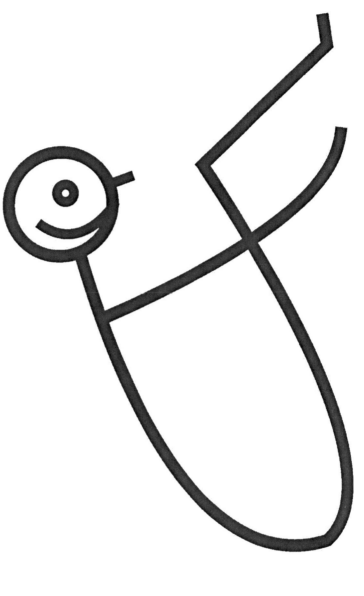

April Merrilee

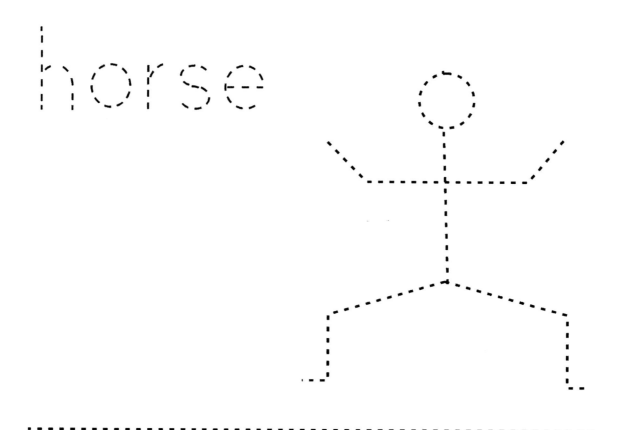

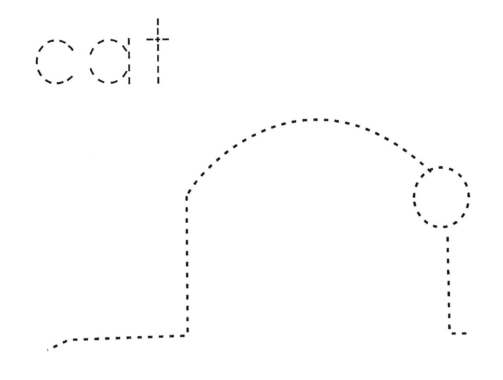

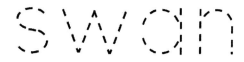

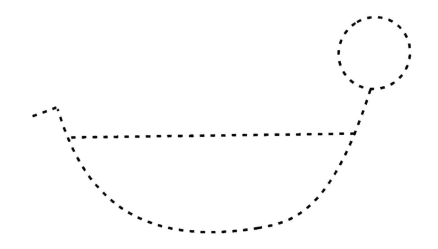

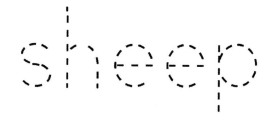

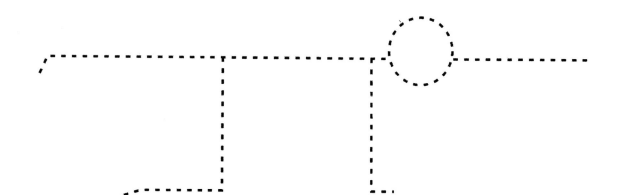

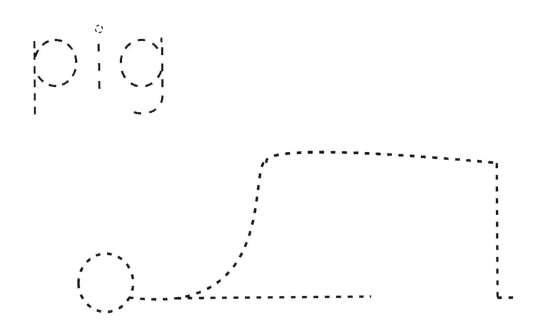

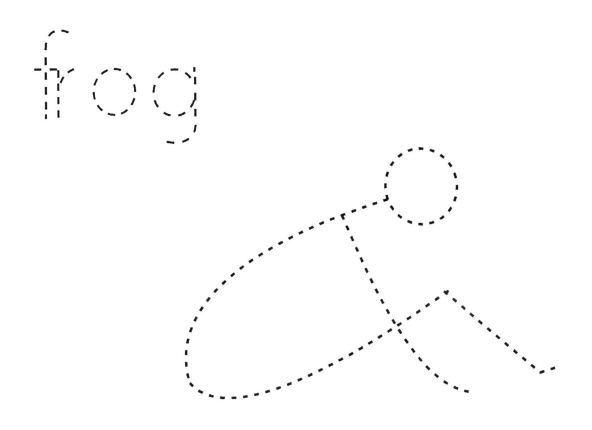

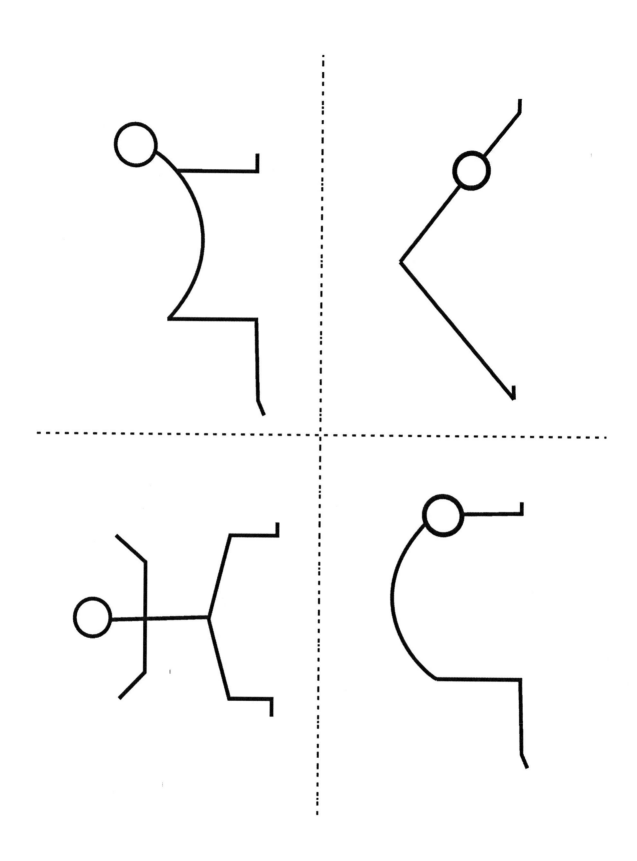

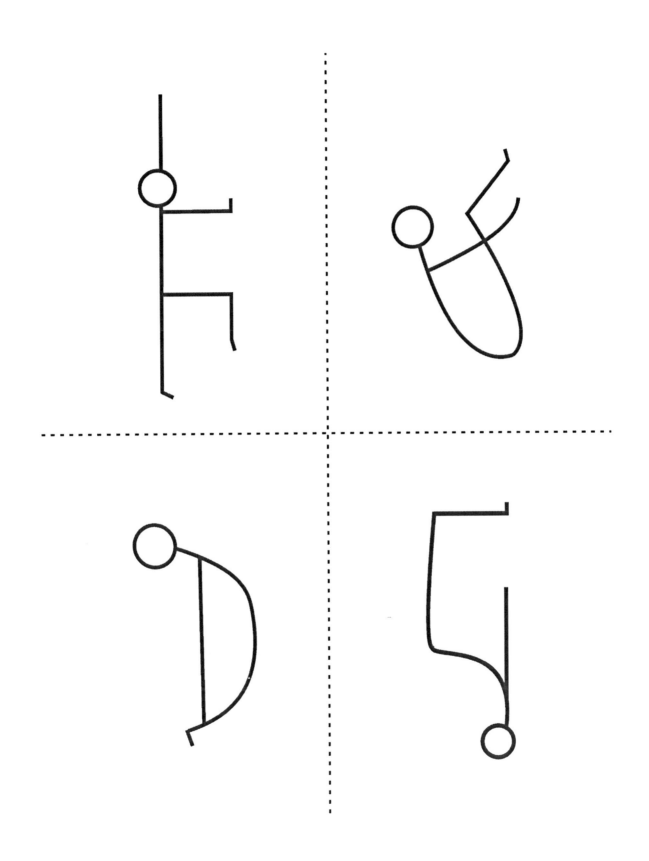

April Merrilee

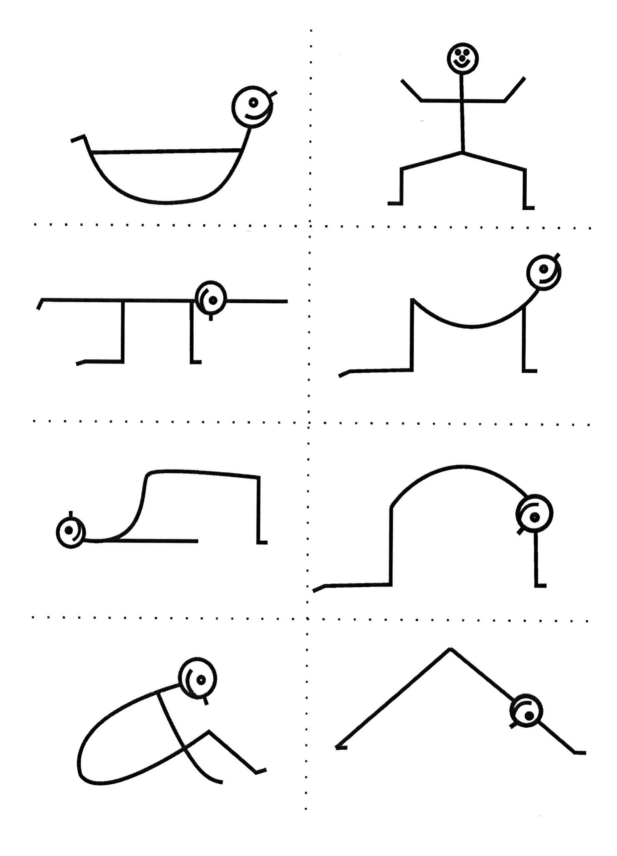

sheep	cow
horse	cat
pig	dog
frog	swan

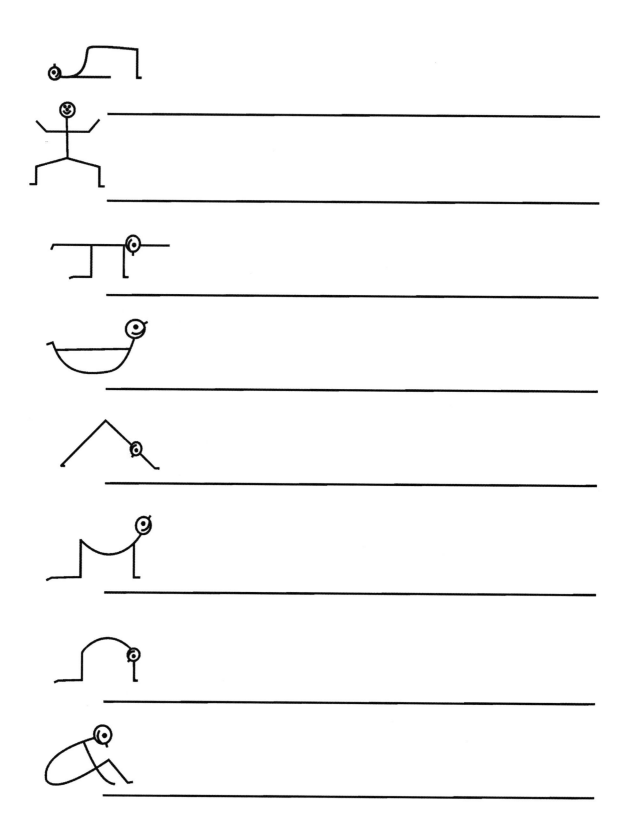

Basic Sentence Worksheet   Mama Duck

Copy these sentences next to the correct drawing on the following page.

The horse is big.

The cow has spots.

The cat is small.

The dog is happy.

The swan can swim.

The sheep is white.

The pig likes mud.

The frog is green.

Challenge Sentence Worksheet: Match and copy next to the correct drawing!

You can feed me corn and slop.

I get to run all around the farm.

I like to chew on hay and carrots.

You can make a blanket with my wool.

I can glide across the water.

I give the farmer my milk.

You can hear me sing at night.

I have whiskers on my face.

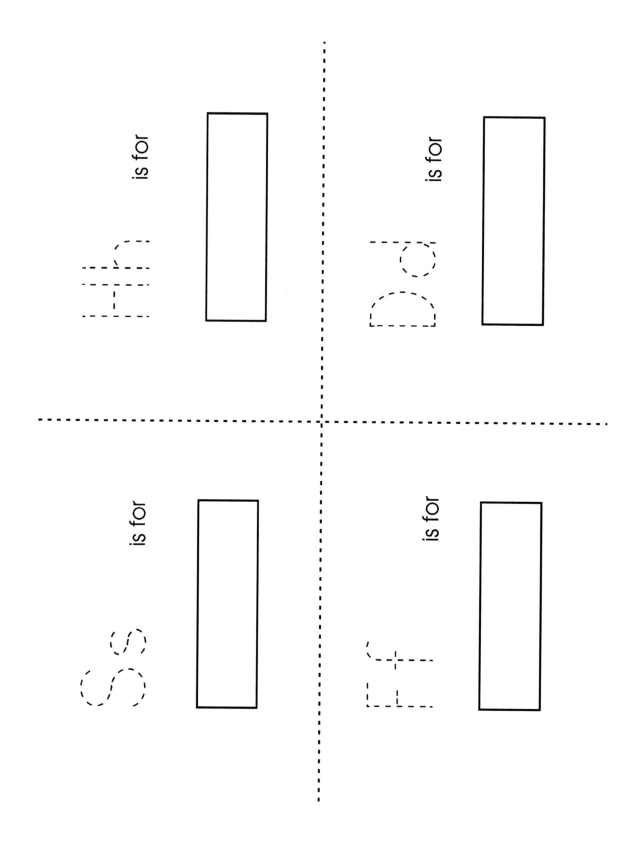

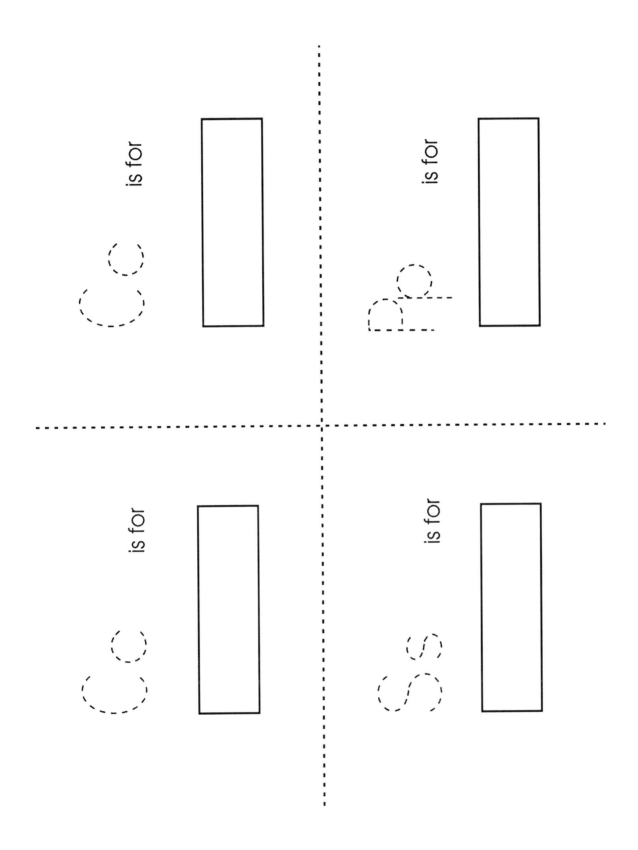

SECTION NINE:

Additional Information

- Schedule a S.M.I.L.Y. workshop in your area
- Order S.M.I.L.Y. CD's -   soundtrack and pose instruction

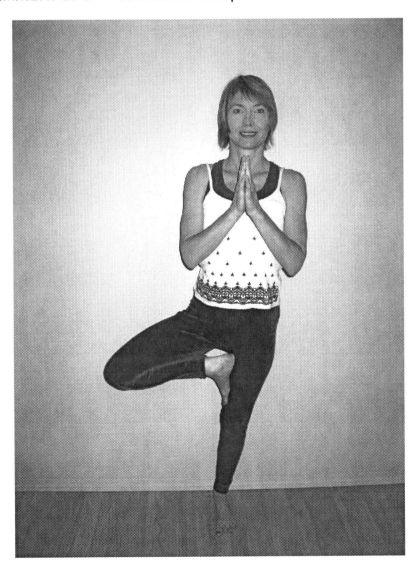

REFERENCES

Asher, J.J., <u>Learning Another Language through Activities: The Complete Teacher's Guide</u>, 6th edition, Sky Oaks, Las Gatos, CA (1996)

Ayres, A. Jean, <u>Sensory Integration and the Child</u>, Western Psychological Services, Los Angeles, CA (1979)

Balzer-Martin, Lynn A., <u>Sensory Integration: Theory, Assessment, Treatment and Screening Program for Young Children</u>, Medical Educational Services, Inc. – Professional Development Network (MEDS-PDN), Eau Claire, WI (2003)

Block, B.A., "Literacy through movement: an organizational approach", <u>Journal of Physical Education, Recreation and Dance</u>, vol 72 (2001)

Buday, E.M., "The effects of signed and spoken words taught with music on sign and speech imitation by children with autism", <u>Journal of Music Therapy</u>, vol 32 (1995)

Cassidy, J. and Standley, J., "The effect of music listening on physiological responses of premature infants in the NICU", <u>Journal of Music Therapy</u>, vol 32 (1995)

Criswell, Eleanor, <u>How Yoga Works: An Introduction to Somatic Yoga</u>, Freeperson Press, Novato, CA (1989)

Gardner, Howard, <u>Frames of Mind: The Theory of Multiple Intelligences</u>, Basic Books, New York, NY, second edition (1992)

Hannaford, C., <u>Smart Moves: Why Learning is Not All in Your Head</u>, Great Ocean Publishers, Arlington, VA (1995)

Jensen, E., <u>Teaching with the Brain in Mind</u>, ASCD, Alexandria, VA (1998)

Jensen, E., <u>The Learning Brain</u>, Turning Point Publishing, Del Mar, CA (1994)

Landy, J and Burridge, K., <u>Fine Motor Skills & Handwriting Activities for The Young Child</u>, The Center for Applied Research in Education, West Nyack, NY (1999)

Levinowitz, Lili M., "The Importance of Music in Early Childhood", <u>General Music Today</u>, Music Educator's National Conference, Fall 1998

Mitchell, D., "The relationship between rhythmic competency and academic performance, University of Florida (2003)

Naveen, et al, "Yoga Breathing Through a Particular Nostril Increases Spatial Memory Scores Without Lateralized Effects", Psychological Reports, vol 81 (1997)

Neuman, S., Copple, C. and Bredekamp, S., Learning to Read and Write: Developmentally Appropriate Practices for Young Children, NAEYC, Washington, D.C. (2000)

Palmer, H., "The Music, Movement and Learning Connection", Young Child, (Sept. 2001)

Pica, R., Moving and Learning Across the Curriculum, Delmar, Clifton Park, NY (1999)

Ratey, J., A User's Guide to the Brain: Perception, Attention and the Four Theaters of the Brain, Vintage Books (2001)

Rauscher, et al, "Music training causes long term enhancement of preschool children's spatial-temporal reasoning", Neurological Research, vol 19 (1997)

Schlag, Gottfried, et al, Nature (1995)

Shatz, C., "The Developing Brain", Scientific American, vol 267:3 (1992)

Shore, R., Rethinking the Brain: New Insights into Early Development, Families and Work Institute, New York (1997)

Sumar, Sonia (1998) Yoga for the Special Child, Special Yoga Publications, Buckingham, Virginia

Sylwester, R., A Biological Brain in a Cultural Classroom: Enhancing Cognitive and Social Development through Collaborative Classroom Management (2001)

Telles, et al (1997) "Comparison of Changes in Autonomic and Respiratory Parameters of Girls After Yoga and Games at a Community Home" in Perceptual and Motor Skills, vol 84, pp 251-257

Telles, et al (1993) "Improvement in Static Motor Performance Following Yogic Training of School Children" in Perceptual and Motor Skills, vol 76, pp 1264-1266

Uma, et al (1989) "The integrated approach of yoga: a therapeutic tool For mentally retarded children: a one year controlled study" in Journal of Mental Deficiency Research, vol 33, pp 415-421

About the Author

April Merrilee received her degree in Occupational Therapy from the University of New Mexico in Albuquerque in 1997 and has remained in the southwest ever since. April has been working as a pediatric O.T. for seven years, serving children of all ages and abilities from infancy through adolescence in school settings and home environments. She has been practicing yoga for 17 years, and has earned four separate teaching certifications including Yoga Therapy and Yoga for the Special Child. April teaches the SMILY program at preschools, elementary schools, day care settings and yoga studios several times a week throughout the year with children ranging in age from 18 months to 9 years. She is available to teach therapists, teachers, parents and caregivers how to lead the SMILY program with children in your area. Feel free to call her toll free number to set up a workshop at your convenience. April currently lives in beautiful Pagosa Springs, Colorado where she enjoys resting in her hammock looking out at the Continental Divide.

ARRANGE FOR A SMILY WORKSHOP
– IN YOUR AREA !!

1 day (7 contact hours); 1 ½ days (11 contact hours) or 2 days (14 hours)

Contact April Merrilee for scheduling:

>Stream of Life Therapeutics, LLC
>P.O. Box 4973
>Pagosa Springs, CO 81157

cell   970-398-0002
toll free   **1-888-276-3716**
website   www.kidsmusicandmovement.com
e-mail   smily@kidsmusicandmovement.com

S.M.I.L.Y. COMPANION C.D.'s
A two CD set providing
* Soundtrack of all 8 S.M.I.L.Y. songs
* Narrated instruction of yoga poses for each routine
* April telling the story for each routine

Call toll free for ordering information: 1-888-276-3716
Visit the website at www.kidsmusicandmovement.com

>Stream of Life Therapeutics, LLC
>P.O. Box 4973
>Pagosa Springs, CO 81157

Thanks so very much for your support.
May you enjoy S.M.I.L.Y. to the fullest!

Printed in the United States
89379LV00002B/47-94/A